JAN MALLO
07835 68(

Lifestyle Medicine Works

Dean Ornish MD, David L. Katz MD,

T. Colin Campbell Ph.D., Bruce Lipton Ph.D.,

Drs. Ayesha and Dean Sherzai, Dr. David Perlmutter,

Joel Fuhrman MD, Neal D. Barnard MD, Ocean Robbins,

Johannes R. Fisslinger LPHCS, Aisling Killoran MA,

Annie Gedye B.Sc., Yasmine Farouk MA, Jane Oelke Ph.D.,

Dr. Tom O'Bryan, Louise Harris, LPHCS,

Bernie Siegel MD, Yeliz Ruzgar B.Sc, LPHCS,

Mohammad Ilyas Yamani, MD, Dr. Kevin Chan

Recorded and transcribed during

the Lifestyle Medicine Summit 2021

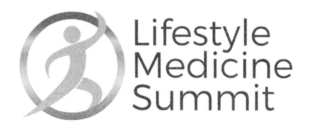

Register for our upcoming global Lifestyle Medicine Summit at

www.lifestylemedicine.io

© 2022 Lifestyle Medicine University Foundation

A 501c3 non-profit organization with a mission to make Lifestyle Medicine and Health Coaching accessible to everyone.

Lifestyle Medicine Works is a trademark of Lifestyle Medicine University Foundation. Lifestyle Prescriptions® is a registered global trademark and can only be used after written approval by the Lifestyle Prescriptions® University.

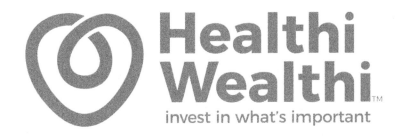

Shouldn't you get "PAID" living healthier, happier, longer, and richer?

Get your Personal 24/7 Health Coach
or build your Health Coaching practice.

Join our Global Movement,
redeem your RXHEAL reward tokens,
and read the book "HealthiWealthi™".

www.healthiwealthi.io.

This book is dedicated to anyone passionately
helping to make Lifestyle Medicine and
Health Coaching accessible to everyone.

A Special Thank You to Bella Donna, for editing,
Yeliz Ruzgar, Dr. Mitra Ray, Loren Lahav, Tony Rodrigues,
and all Lifestyle Medicine Summit Expert Speakers,
for leading the way.

Table of Contents

Chapter One   1

Johannes R. Fisslinger MA, LPHCS - Improving Health Outcomes. Fixing Healthcare. Saving Billions. Creating 100,000 Jobs – A No-Brainer BIG PROPOSAL!

Chapter Two   8

Dean Ornish MD - Lifestyle Medicine Brand New Evidence

Chapter Three   28

David L. Katz MD - Is Lifestyle Medicine the Best Medicine We Have Got?

Chapter Four   44

T. Colin Campbell Ph.D. - Nutrition Reformation and Renaissance (The China Study)

Chapter Five   60

Bruce Lipton Ph.D. - Medicine, Consciousness, and Healing

Chapter Six   81

Drs. Ayesha and Dean Sherzai – Building Healthy Brains

Chapter Seven   95

Dr. David Perlmutter – Alzheimer's, Dementia, and Brain Health

v

Chapter Eight 110

Joel Fuhrman MD – Autoimmune, Inflammatory Bowel, Diabetes, Heart Disease, and More

Chapter Nine 126

Neal D. Barnard MD – Diabetes, Hot Flashes, and Thyroid: Nutrition Interventions

Chapter Ten 139

Ocean Robbins - The Science of Behavior Change (How to Influence People to Change Their Diets!)

Chapter Eleven 155

Johannes R. Fisslinger MA, LPHCS - How to Prescribe Lifestyle Medicine in 3 Minutes: Without Changing Your Workflow or Increasing Expenses

Chapter Twelve 171

Johannes R. Fisslinger MA, LPHCS - Organ-Mind-Brain Anatomy™, the 6 Root-Causes and the Art and Science of Self-Healing

Chapter Thirteen 181

Aisling Killoran - Psychosocial Stressors and Infertility (New Research)

Chapter Fourteen 192

Annie Gedye B.Sc., LPHCS - The 9 Points and Phases of Chronic Symptoms and the Autonomic Nervous System

Chapter Fifteen — 204

Yasmine Farouk MA, LPHCS - The Emotion-Body Roller Coaster

Chapter Sixteen — 216

Jane Oelke ND, Ph.D. - Fibromyalgia, Chronic Pain, Emotions, and Limiting Beliefs

Chapter Seventeen — 229

Dr. Tom O'Bryan - How Food Choices Determine a Better Way for Your Health

Chapter Eighteen — 237

Louise Harris - Helping Children and Families with Neurological Disorders, Anxiety, and Sleep Issues

Chapter Nineteen — 248

Bernie Siegel MD - Stories of Wisdom. Healthcare Reimagined

Chapter Twenty — 258

Yeliz Ruzgar B.Sc., LPHCS - Life Purpose, Wellness and Longevity (Science of Being)

Chapter Twenty-One — 274

Dr. M.I. Yamani - #1 Medical Error: Failure To Diagnose and Value-Based-Care.

Chapter Twenty-Two — 284

Dr. Kevin Chan - Secrets to successful Lifestyle Medicine Practice

Chapter One

Johannes R. Fisslinger MA, LPHCS - Improving Health Outcomes. Fixing Healthcare. Saving Billions. Creating 100,000 Jobs – A No-Brainer BIG PROPOSAL!

Johannes is the founder of Lifestyle Prescriptions® University, HealthiWealthi™ RXHEAL Coach Platform & Ecosystem, author of "The 6-Root-Causes of All Symptoms", and host of the "Lifestyle Medicine Summit and "Health Coach Summit. ↗ lifestylemedicine.io

If you've heard the first time about Lifestyle Medicine and Health Coaching then the expert speakers in this book will clearly demonstrate that there's a solution to the Chronic Disease Pandemic we're experiencing right now.

Before we dive into the why and how of Lifestyle Medicine I feel it's important to start this book with 2 solutions that'll transform healthcare, guaranteed.

Here they are:

If you are a health and life lover, there are two questions that can make a huge difference in your life and in the lives of millions around the planet.

Ask your doctor and healthcare provider:

"Do you offer lifestyle medicine?"

"Do you prescribe lifestyle medicine and health coaching?"

Just think about that for a second and visualize how this could play out. If you don't ask, you won't ever know if they offer root-cause solutions for chronic health issues. No matter who your healthcare provider or nutritionist is, or whatever other specialists you come in contact with, ask them.

If we keep asking these questions, healthcare providers will adjust to the demand and start implementing these new chronic disease solution strategies.

Why?

Because Lifestyle Medicine Works!

But actually, this is not my BIG PROPOSAL.

Here it is:

Improving Health Outcomes. Fixing Healthcare. Saving Billions. Creating 100,000 Jobs – A No-Brainer Strategy!

It's been said many times: Follow the money ... and I believe it also applies to our healthcare system.

Let me share with you why 100,000 full-time and well-trained health coaches in the US will fix the US healthcare system, save $ BILLIONS in healthcare costs, why it's not a dream but a necessity and a reality we'll see sooner than we think.

Here we go:

The U.S. healthcare costs have skyrocketed to $3.65 Trillion in 2018 and projections indicate an increase by at least 5.5% annually over the next decade. This number is so huge that you really have to see it numerically:

$3,650,000,000,000

($3.65 Trillion)

Just think about this: US healthcare spending accounted for 17.9 percent of GDP which is over $10,739 per person. [1]

We also know that over 80% of today's healthcare costs are connected to non-communicable (chronic) lifestyle diseases like obesity, diabetes, heart disease, pain, Alzheimer's, Anxiety, Depression, and other auto-immune disorders. [2]

Traditional medicine solutions are mostly focused on "managing" these very expensive conditions and even new advances in technology won't change this downward spiral because they are not designed or meant to address the root-causes and reverse chronic symptoms.

There is a vast agreement between health professionals, governments, and patients that this is not sustainable and more importantly that we won't solve the healthcare crisis without new innovative ideas.

Now, here is my specific proposal:

We invest in Lifestyle Medicine Doctors and Health Coaches on a national and global scale!

Hear me out.

Extensive research shows that by preventing chronic disease we obviously improve health outcomes and save healthcare costs. For example, studies have shown that the reduction of bypass surgery and stents can save $30,000 per patient in the first year alone, therefore, cutting healthcare costs by 50% in the first year.

---

[1] https://fortune.com/2019/02/21/us-health-care-costs-2/ and https://www.ncbi.nlm.nih.gov/pmc/articles/PMC6211719

[2] www.www.fightchronicdisease.org/sites/default/files/docs/GrowingCrisisofChronic DiseaseintheUSfactsheet_81009.pdf.

It's safe to estimate that healthcare cost savings of 2-10% annually are absolutely possible. [3]

WOW, that's a whopping $73-365 BILLION in SAVINGS.

Depending on some variables and current annual healthcare expenses of $3,650,000,000,000 we save:

$73,000,000,000 (2% or $73 Billion saved)

$182,500,000,000 (5% or $182 Billion saved)

$365,000,000,000 (10% or $365 Billion saved)

Let's be conservative and take the next step in this new **Healthcare 3.0** model based on Prevention, Lifestyle Medicine and Health Coach focused healthcare model.

How could we create a win-win-win situation with new high-paying, fulfilling jobs being created, the strain on current health professionals eased, and most importantly, the health and productivity of people improved?

Stay with me ... here's how:

- 328,000,000 people living in the US
- 120,000,000 (120 Million) households
- 25,000,000 high-risk households that need coaching (20%)
- 250 households (about 1,000 individuals) are supported by one health coach

100,000 health coaches are needed to coach up to 100 million individuals.

Each health coach receives approx. $73,000 annual income / reimbursement.

---

[3] 3) https://www.ncbi.nlm.nih.gov/pubmed/9860380

This means we need to invest ONLY 0.2% of the annual healthcare cost into prevention ($7.3 Billion) and based on estimates, we'll SAVE 2% of the annual healthcare cost annually ($73 Billion).

That's absolutely astounding!

Now, you might ask, what are these health coaches going to do?

Because health coaches are paid properly they can focus 100% of their time and skills to help chronic disease patients shift their unhealthy habits to

- Eat better
- Exercise more
- Stress less
- Love more.

Each health coach is responsible for supporting his/her patients using:

- Health Coaching Group Sessions
- Working with individual or families in personal consultations
- Prescribing micro-habit Lifestyle Medicine or Root-Cause Lifestyle Prescriptions®
- Engaging clients to establish healthy habits
- Providing support and helping clients overcome challenges

Naturally, the best part is that addressing the root-causes will not just help manage symptoms, it will help reverse them, quality of life and relationships will dramatically improve, and we'll save billions in healthcare costs which can be re-invested.

Just think about what we could do with these $$$:

- Re-invested into Lifestyle Medicine research
- Lower healthcare costs for businesses and families
- Repay our national depth
- The possibilities are endless ...

Let's summarize:

We invest 0.2% of current annual healthcare expenditure into 100,000 highly qualified and efficient Lifestyle Medicine Doctors & Health Coaches working with 250 households each, improving health outcomes, productivity & quality of life of up to 100 million people, and save billions in healthcare costs in return.

Sounds like a no-brainer to me!

The only problem is that unless we take action and demand new innovations in healthcare based on prevention and lifestyle medicine it won't happen.

Here's a solution:

SHARE this book to everyone you know especially health professionals, insurance, and government decision-makers!

DEMAND CHOICES.

Ask your doctor to prescribe Lifestyle Medicine and be referred to a health coach. If NOT you can always find a new doctor or clinic, right!

* Here's my disclaimer: Please don't beat up on me, if some of these numbers are not 100% correct. My point is to demonstrate that transforming and creating Healthcare 3.0 based on Prevention, Lifestyle Medicine, and Health Coaching is possible.

But do we have the will and political strength to take this step?

Enjoy this book and the wisdom of global leaders in Lifestyle Medicine and Health Coaching.

In case you might ask yourself: This is exciting in theory but there is no way this can be implemented nationally.

Well, it's actually being done, right now.

Check www.healthiwealthi.io.

Chapter Two

Dean Ornish MD - Lifestyle Medicine Brand New Evidence

Considered the "Father of Lifestyle Medicine." Founder and President of the nonprofit Preventive Medicine Research Institute in Sausalito, California. Clinical Professor of Medicine at the University of California, San Francisco. Bestselling Author.
↗ Ornish.com

Lifestyle medicine is using lifestyle changes, not only to help prevent disease, which we all know, but to treat, and often even reverse it. In many ways, the biggest obstacle that I find with lifestyle medicine is the idea that for many people, they think, "Oh, diet and lifestyle, that's kind of boring. How powerful could that be?"

I think our unique contribution has been to use these very high-tech, expensive, state-of-the-art scientific measures to prove how powerful these very low-tech and low-cost interventions can be.

Our method of study over the years has been the same for all these different disease and health issues.

Our whole foods, plant-based diet:

- Is low in fats, refined sugars and refined carbs
- Includes various meditation and yoga-based stress management techniques
- Incorporates personalized exercise
- Encourages psychosocial support
- Helps people feel better, live longer, lose weight, and gain health

Reduced to its essence:

- Eating well
- Moving more
- Stressing less
- Loving more

The more diseases we study, the more scientific evidence we have of how powerful these simple changes are, and how quickly we can measure improvements in how people feel, maintain, and exist day-to-day.

A panel of experts at US News and World Report rates us every year just as they rate hospitals and medical centers. And for ten years since 2011, including this year, they rated the *Ornish Diet* as number one for heart health; which I think is a nice vote of confidence.

What differentiates our work from so many others is that we have 44 years of work published in leading peer-reviewed journals showing that these lifestyle changes cannot only help prevent, but often stop and even reverse the progression of the most common chronic diseases and include one of the first demonstrated randomized trials that heart disease can be reversed or early-stage prostate cancer.

Our research shows that lifestyle changes can reverse the progression of:

- Type 2 diabetes
- High blood pressure
- Autoimmune diseases
- High cholesterol
- Obesity
- Cellular aging
- Gene expression

You may wonder how simple lifestyle changes can have such far-reaching implications? Or, how can one program be a fit for all without personalization? Our studies show that a fundamental program can be the same yet help with so many different conditions.

I wrote a book called UnDo It! with my wife who has been my partner for 22 years. We put forth a new unifying theory inspired by one of our favorite quotes from Albert Einstein. It is the first quote in my book, "If you can't explain it simply, you don't understand it well enough." We've attempted to reduce healthy lifestyle changes to its essence.

The unifying theory how these same lifestyle changes can help prevent and reverse so many different chronic diseases is that most diseases are not as different as we've been told.

As I've worked with different diseases, diagnoses, and treatments, I discovered the manifestations are the results of the same underlying biological mechanisms.

Commonalities in each of these genes and mechanisms include:

- Chronic inflammation
- Overstimulation of the sympathetic nervous system
- Changes in immune function, and the microbiome
- Oxidative stress
- Apoptosis (programmed cell death)
- Angiogenesis and telomere changes
- Gene expressions

These are directly influenced by:

- What we eat
- How we respond to stress
- Amount of exercise

- Love in our lives
- Social and personal support

All of this helps explain why we often find the same person with a collection of diseases, issues, and health imbalances including:

- Weight problems
- High blood pressure
- High cholesterol
- Type 2 diabetes
- Heart disease

We can see again, the same diseases manifesting in different ways, as well as the same manifestations from different diseases.

This helps explain why, as an example, T. Colin Campbell's, The China Project, concluded one of the most comprehensive nutritional studies every undertaken:

"China at that time presented researchers with a unique opportunity. The Chinese population tended to live in the same area all their lives and to consume the same diets unique to each region. Their diets (low in fat and high in dietary fiber and plant material) also were in stark contrast to the rich diets of the Western countries. The truly plant-based nature of the rural Chinese diet gave researchers a chance to compare plant-based diets with animal-based diets."

The Center for Disease Control (CDC) even released a report that lifestyle changes can reduce the risk of chronic disease, stating that better dietary options, as well as increased physical activity and weight management has many benefits.

Proof again that the same lifestyle changes affect so many different aspects of our health and lives.

Statistically, diabetes is at an all-time high in the United States. From 1998 to 2008, the increase of diabetes was 90% as reported at medicalnewstoday.com. Diabetic Research online reported in 2018 that 10.2% of the U.S. population or an estimated 26.8 million people have diabetes.

A 2022 report by EHA Today (European Hematology Association online) entitled 1 in 3 American Adults has Pre-diabetes Millions at Risk for Type 2 Diabetes says, "Once people are made aware of their condition, they are more likely to make the necessary long-term lifestyle changes, such as eating healthier, managing weight, and being active, that can help prevent or delay the onset of type 2 diabetes."

Ongoing research and statistics show how powerful simple changes are and what a tremendous impact they can have on people's lives.

COVID 2020 IMPACT

I also want to take a moment to talk about COVID-19 and lifestyle since this is obviously on everyone's mind since 2020. We all know that people with chronic diseases have a much higher risk of getting COVID, being hospitalized, and dying from it.

A September 2021, study at Harvard Medical School states:

In a study of close to 600,000 people, Jordi Merino, a research associate at the Diabetes Unit and Center for Genomic Medicine at Massachusetts General Hospital (MGH), concluded, "Previous reports suggest that poor diet is a common trait in groups disproportionately affected by the pandemic, but there is a lack of data on the relationship between diet and COVID-19 risk and severity." [4]

And in yet another study, GreenQueen, an online health newsletter reported in June of 2021, **"Plant-based diets are linked to 73% lower risk of severe Covid-19, new global study finds."**

Their study involved 2,800 healthcare professionals from six different countries as part of the Survey Healthcare Globus Network. [5]

This same study also showed that those, "… practicing a low-carbohydrate, high-protein diet had nearly four-times the odds of moderate to severe infections from Covid-19", based on an online survey conducted between July and September 2020.

We can conclude then that just avoiding exposure to a virus – mask wearing, vaccinating, avoiding crowds, and so on, is not the best approach to staying well. How our bodies partake in functional lifestyle is the best choice for overall health and wellness.

Facts:

- People who are sedentary have more than double the risk of being hospitalized or dying due to COVID.
- Overweight people have triple the risk of hospitalization, ICU admission, and death, especially younger people.

The underlying theory of lifestyle medicine is summarized in this cartoon I have been sharing for over forty years now. This is

---

[4] https://dailyzhealthpress.com/diet-could-affect-coronavirus-risk-according-to-mgh-study-harvard-gazette/

[5] https://www.greenqueen.com.hk/plant-based-diets-linked-73-lower-risk-of-severe-covid-19-new-global-study-finds/

as true today as it was years ago. Modern medicine seems to spend so much time mopping up the floor, without turning off the faucet.

CHRONIC HEALTH ISSUES

Drugs and surgery can be lifesaving when used appropriately in acute care. In the case of a heart attack, drugs and surgery can be lifesaving. But we always want to ask the question, "What caused the problem in the first place?"

The results of illnesses are the lifestyle choices that we make each day. What I'm continually impressed by is that if we treat an illness with lifestyle changes oftentimes our bodies have this remarkable capacity to begin healing. The body even responses more quickly when treating causes rather than symptoms. Everything was thought impossible before we began doing it. And to me, one of the benefits of doing research and why I spend so much of my life doing what I do is that it can raise awareness and redefine what's possible. By doing so, it can give many people new hope and new choices.

In 1977, when I was a second-year medical student, I took a year off to do a one-month intervention with 10 men and women in a hotel for a month. Eight of the ten people got better.

I did a second study after finishing medical school and after just three and a half weeks, we showed improvements in the ability of the heart to pump blood. This study was published in the Journal of the American Medical Association and referenced in the February 2009, issue of Today's Dietitian online.

"Ornish gives a snapshot of his scientific findings on the lifestyle program, starting with a pilot study of 10 patients in 1977 showing that his program made an improvement in blood flow to the heart in only one month. In 1983, The Journal of the American Medical Association published a randomized,

14

controlled trial that showed the heart's ability to pump blood improved significantly in only one month.

The first randomized trial that demonstrated even severe coronary artery blockages could reverse in only one year was published in The Lancet in 1990. Five-year findings were published in The Journal of the American Medical Association in 1998, indicating that there was even more reversal after five years than after one year. Ornish reports that the five-year results showed an average improvement to the heart of more than 300% and 2.5 times fewer cardiac events."

After medical school I went on to Boston to do my medical residency and fellowship; then moved to San Francisco. There I began the most definitive study called the "Lifestyle Heart Trials." In the earlier years we used quantitative arteriography to measure blockages in the arteries. Later, cardiac Positron Emission Tomography (PET) scans were used to measure blood flow and cardiac issues.

With our scanning and tracking we were able to see that arteries naturally seemed to clog over time, thus resulting in a history of heart disease.

With the information we could collect with our equipment, we then observed in an experimental group, a reversal of arterial blockages in one year with lifestyle changes. The result of this study is published in the July 1990, Lancet article, can lifestyle changes reverse coronary heart disease? [6]

Even more impressive, after five years, a 400% improvement in blood flow was measured in PET scans as evidence of heart-health improvement with lifestyle changes. This is noted in an Ornish Lifestyle online publication Healthways, dated 2017

---

[6] https://www.thelancet.com/journals/lancet/article/PII0140-6736(90)91656-U/fulltext

This article states:

"Overall, there was a 400% statistically significant and clinically significant improvement in myocardial perfusion in the experimental group when compared to the randomized control group after five years. 99% of patients in the experimental group of the Lifestyle Heart Trial showed improvement or no change in their cardiac PET scans after 5 years. In contrast, 45% of controls had worsening perfusion defects, 50% showed no change, and only 5% improved."

This shows that a modest increase in the radius causes an exponential improvement in blood flow. Not only did a few patients show improvement, but 99% of the patients were able to stop or reverse their heart disease as measured by PET scans. Only 5% of the randomized control group improved. We've published this in a December 1998, JAMA paper. [7]

This researched confirmed that the more people changed their lifestyle, at any age, there is improvement. This is a very empowering realization.

I was involved with a man who had a massive heart attack and was told the only thing that could save his life was a heart transplant. While waiting for a doctor, he went through my UCLA program for reversing heart disease so he would be in better shape for the heart transplant. As a result, he got so much better than he didn't need the heart transplant. Which route seems more appealing- a heart transplant or a healthy life with less stress and more love in it?

Here is what he had to say:

---

[7] https://jamanetwork.com/journals/jama/fullarticle/188274

"The situation I'm describing here is an internal medicine doctor who started a new chapter in his life with his wife. Moving to Lake Arrowhead, we just opened a private practice office. After all, our kids went to college and we could relocate and just as this was ramping up, we had a horrible car accident that precipitated a heart attack. That dropped my cardiac functioning down to 50% of what it should have been. This resulted in intractable chest pain, angina, trouble breathing, inability to walk from room to room, or even go upstairs without being carried. I was offered a heart transplant as the only way to stay alive.

At the 11th hour, I entered the Ornish program which provided me with an entire paradigm shift concerning stress management, exercise, diet, and nutrition, and despite not believing in it myself and having other physicians who did not believe in it either, it worked. Beyond my wildest dreams, I'm now able to exercise moderately, I can work full time, I can live and breathe at 6000 feet. Our quality of life is better than it was before."

We then found that the same lifestyle changes that work with heart disease could slow, stop, or reverse, the progression of early-stage prostate cancer. This prompted a study with the Chair of Urology at UCSF, Dr. Peter Carroll, and the person who was chair of Urology at Memorial Sloan Kettering Cancer Center in New York.

At the time, we started with men who had biopsy-proven prostate cancer, and who elected to do what was called" watchful waiting." This was so we could then randomize and have a nonintervention control group. This cannot be done with most forms of cancer because most people get treated right away. We found that Prostate-Specific Antigen (PSA) levels went up or got worse than the control group. The differences were highly significant. And they occurred again in direct proportion to the degree of lifestyle changes. The more people improved their lifestyle, the lower their PSA. When we added their serum to a standard line of prostate tumor cells, using a tissue culture at Bill Aronson's lab at UCLA, it resulted in the tumor growth being inhibited by 70%, versus only 9% in the control group.

In a subset of patients, we used Magnetic Resonance (MR) spectroscopy to measure the tumor activity. We noted that as the tumors diminished, the PSA went down. None of the experimental group patients needed surgery, radiation, or chemotherapy, during the first year. Six of the control group patients however did.

This was an extraordinary study showing that any positive lifestyle changes can stop or reverse the progression of early-stage prostate cancer.

In another study with Harvard Physicians Health, it was found that men who ate a mostly Western diet had a 250% higher risk of prostate cancer-related deaths a 67% increased risk of death from any cause. Again, these are all the same diseases manifesting in different ways. [8]

Study after study confirms that whole food, plant-based diets improve all health issues. This is a theme that I keep coming back to. When you move from a typical American or Western diet to a whole food, plant-based diet, essentially a vegetarian or vegan diet that's low in fat and sugar, you are decreasing your risk of all harmful health issues.

We participated in another study done with Craig Venter, who was the first geneticist to decode the human genome. We found that when you positively change your diet, over 500 genes can be impacted in just three months. Often people have been told or will think, "Oh, I've got bad genes, there's nothing I can do about it."

---

[8] https://www.health.harvard.edu/cancer/can-diet-help-fight-prostate-cancer

In fact, there's a lot you can do. Not blaming but empowering yourself is a good starting point. If you think you are just a victim of your bad genes, what can you do, right?

We also found that the genes called the Rat Sarcoma Virus (RAS) oncogenes, those likely to produce prostate, breast, and colon cancer, were turned off. We used a heatmap for this detection. Heatmaps are used to show expressions of specific genes. Red indicates that the gene is turned on, and green indicates that the gene is turned off.

This research confirmed that our genes are not our fate. If you're willing to make positive lifestyle changes, even if your family history predisposes you to a condition like heart disease, it just means you need to make bigger changes to help prevent illness from happening.

We've also done another study with Elizabeth Blackburn. In 2009, Blackburn was awarded the Nobel Prize in Medicine for discovering telomeres. She is the world leader in telomere research. Her and her research team conducted investigations through clinical and human studies. They determined that telomeres protect the ends of our chromosomes from fusing into each other and allow chromosome ends to attach to the nuclear envelope which prevents you from aging.

Based on this discovery, we now know that as our telomeres shorten over time, and thus our life expectancy does also. The risk of premature death from so many diseases goes up proportionately. We found that for the first time when people made our recommended lifestyle changes, the telomerase, as well as the enzyme that repairs and lengthens telomeres, went up by 30%.

We've also learned that over time, telomeres can get longer. This was the first study to show that intervention can lengthen

19

telomeres. Counter to this, telomeres shortened in the control group. When this information was published, The Lancet editor sent out a press release worldwide. The press release said that the study reveals first-ever data indicating that positive lifestyle changes may reverse aging at the cellular level. I believe this is such a great discovery, especially as I get older. So again, we find significant correlation between positive lifestyle changes, telomere health, and human longevity. [9]

BRAIN HEALTH

Something as simple as eating five or more fruits and vegetables a day reduces your risk of cognitive impairment by almost half. Molecular Nutrition and Food Research found that adding fruits, vegetables, and other plant-based foods to your diet could help reduce risk of cognitive decline. [10]

Many other studies show that with people over 65, just eating lots of vegetables reduces dementia by 38%. Something as simple as having omega- fatty3 acids that you find in flaxseed oil, algae-based oil, or fish oil, can reduce your risk of Alzheimer's by 60%. I assure you, if a drug came out that could do that, it would be a multibillion-dollar drug.

It is quite simple. What is bad for your heart is bad for your brain. Saturated fat and trans fats can more than double the risk of developing Alzheimer's disease. Whereas meditation helps slow it down.

Multiple studies have been done with brains of people who meditate versus those who don't. Study after study confirms the fact that meditators have younger brains. One study stated, "When

---

[9] https://mitpress.mit.edu/books/elizabeth-blackburn-and-story-telomeres

https://www.nobelprize.org/prizes/medicine/2009/press-release/

[10] https://onlinelibrary.wiley.com/doi/10.1002/mnfr.202100606

researchers at UCLA compared the brains of meditators to non-meditators, they found that meditator's brains were almost a decade younger by the time people reach their mid-50s." [11]

For anyone who dealing with Alzheimer's, sadly, we have not seen much progress in the research in the past 40 years.

I am currently in the middle of the first randomized trial to see if our recommended lifestyle changes may slow, stop, or even reverse the progression of early-stage Alzheimer's disease. I can't say anything about what we're finding yet, but I'm hopeful.

Our hypothesis is a more intensive one that's been looked at in the past, as we expect to confirm ways to stop or even reverse dementia. As Benjamin Franklin said, "An ounce of prevention is worth a pound of cure."

NOTE: We are still recruiting patients for our study. If you have any interest and live in the U.S, go to pmi.org. It has all the information, and everything is done for free, including 21 meals a week for patients and their spouses or caregivers for the 40 weeks of the intervention.

OPTIMAL EATING HABITS

Let's talk about what an optimal way of eating is. There is a lot of nutritional advice available in recent years showing that the healthiest diet is that of eating plants, fruits, vegetables, whole grains, and legumes in their natural forms.

These foods are low is harmful components while high in protective factors, phytochemicals, bioflavonoids, carotenoids, retinas, isoflavones, and lycopene, which help to starve any cancer and improve heart disease. What we include in our diet is as important as what we exclude. For the greatest benefits, eat

---

[11] https://www.mindful.org/meditators-younger-brains

food as close as possible to its natural form, as well as foods with little or no processing.

The bad fats- hydrogenated fats, saturated fats, and trans fats should be avoided as much as possible.

The good fats- four grams a day of omega-3 fatty acids provide one gram a day of healthy DHA (Docosahexaenoic acid) and EPA (Eicosapentaenoic acid.) Organic is of course better for you because it has fewer endocrine disrupters, insecticides, and so on. And it tastes better. DHA and EPA are the most potent types of omega-3 fatty acids which benefit heart and brain health, and also increase immune function.

Broccoli is a quality source of natural omega-3 fatty acids. Many people are surprised to find how good it tastes if you steam it. It's delicious and is a good substitute for your intake of sugar and refined carbs. Other vegetables high in omega-3 fatty acids are- spinach, Brussel sprouts, purslane, and lefty greens.

It's not just one change of habit that helps make a difference in your health, but a lot of changes that can make the biggest difference.

I am staying away from the fat versus carbs debate, and that it's the animal protein, independent of the fat and carbs, that may also be a problem.

One study, led by researchers at Harvard T.H. Chan School of Public Health states:

"... findings suggest that replacing (saturated) fats with healthier fats, whole grains, and plant proteins may reduce coronary heart disease risk." And "Eating an overall healthy diet that includes fruits, vegetables, whole grains, vegetable cooking oils rich in polyunsaturated fats, nuts, legumes, fish and low-fat dairy is recommended."

Animal protein increases premature mortality from all causes, whereas plant protein is associated with lower mortality. When you replace animal protein with plant protein you are lowering your risk of many factors.

Another study done at Cleveland Clinic, looked at trimethylamine-N-oxide (TMAO), a risk factor for heart disease. This study found Trimethyllysine (TML), a precursor to TMAO was highest in Atkins-type diets, moderate in the Mediterranean diet, and lowest on what was referred to as "a side order."

It's worth pointing out that with all the different diet information available that the only diet that's been proven in randomized trials to reverse the progression of heart disease, is the one that we've been talking about - a whole foods, plant-based diet, low in fats and sugar.

On the other hand, a low carb diet, the Atkins, Paleo, and the ketogenic diet, are all associated with a 30% increase of all causes of mortality and a 51% higher cardiovascular mortality. This is from the New England Journal of Medicine.

ARTERIES HEALTH

What happens to your arteries on different diets? In the plant-based diet that I recommend, they stay clean. On a Western diet, they are partially clogged due to high fat, high protein, and a low carb diet. Even with the Western diet, if weight goes down, the arteries can stay clogged. This is what confuses a lot of people. Most Americans, as well as Europeans, consume way too much sugar and refined carbs. There are clearly many benefits to reducing these.

However, replacing carbs and sugar with no protein is not a good idea. Replacing them with whole foods, fruits, vegetables, whole grains, legumes, and soy products is optimal, providing healthy protein.

A high animal protein diet is known to increase health risk factors, evidenced by low numbers of "circulating endothelial progenitor cells." These are like little Pac-Man cells that nibble away at keeping your arteries clean. Also shown with this high animal protein diet is an elevated number of esterified fatty acids which cause inflammation and increases atherosclerosis.

To add a little dark humor ... the cows being led off to the slaughterhouse are saying, "My only consolation is that by eating us, they're killing themselves."

THE COST OF HEALTH "CARE"

A protein, plant-based diet is not only medically effective and cost-efficient, but it turns out that 5% of people account for 50 to 80% of all health care costs. This is according to a 2016 report from the U. S. Department of Health and Human Services. Also reported, is that 22.8% of health care spending goes to just 1% of the population. This small group is referred to as "The Super Users." Do you see the relationship here between health and healthcare costs?

If the protein, plant-based diet could target those people who are already sick, we can slowly lower health care costs for all.

In the past, we did a study with Mutual of Omaha, where they found that 80% of the people who were told "you need a stent or a bypass" were able to safely avoid it by changing their lifestyle going on my program instead. Mutual of Omaha saved almost $30,000 per patient in the first year. It's important to show cost savings in the first year because insurance companies in the United States know that a third of people change companies and change jobs every year. Their logic was, "If it's going to take longer than a year, why should we spend our money for some future benefit that someone else will get?" Showing costs in the first year became a game-changer.

We did a second study with Highmark Blue Cross Blue Shield which not only covered my program but provided it at 26 sites in West Virginia, Nebraska, and Pennsylvania. Information on the study, as well as encouragement to subscribers was written about in a member magazine dated 2006. [12]

I saw a cartoon once that said, "I can operate, or you can go on a strict diet." The patient replies, "You better operate, my insurance doesn't cover a strict diet." We see that the medical profession with good science isn't enough to make a difference in people's lives when insurance coverage is not aligned with health.

After 16 years of review with Medicare, they created a new benefit category to cover my program for reversing heart disease. It's called "intensive cardiac rehabilitation."

Many other insurance companies are now covering this as well. This was a huge game-changer, and now offers a healthy option available to people who need it most. I didn't want this to be just for concierge medicine.

In October of 2020, due to COVID, Medicare began reimbursing for my program when done via Zoom. This allows us to reach people wherever they live. It helps reduce health disparities and health inequities. We can reach people in rural areas, minorities, and other people who wouldn't have access to this otherwise. We're hoping that they'll continue to do this. Our approach is a team approach. We have a doctor, a nurse, a meditation teacher, exercise physiologists, dietitians, psychologists, and whoever else is necessary. People meet for four-hour sessions, twice a week for nine weeks. Their programs consist of exercise, a meditation support group, and a lecture with a group meal.

---

[12] https://www.highmarkbcbswv.com/PDFFiles/Healthy-Lifestyles-Spring-2006.pdf

When a program is reimbursable, it seems sustainable. What we learned from this program was that 94% of the people finished all 72 hours. The success rate is higher than people's adherence to taking statins or other drugs. The reason is, when people make lifestyle changes, they start noticing immediate results and feel better about themselves. It reframes the reason for making these changes from fear of dying—which is not sustainable—to joy, pleasure, love, and feeling good, which are like the man mentioned earlier who was able to avoid heart surgery.

He was a man who couldn't walk across the street without getting chest pain, had to be carried up to his room, couldn't make love with his wife without getting chest pain, couldn't go back to work, couldn't do much of anything, then within just a few weeks, he can do all those things.

We are led to believe that we'll miss things like eating junk food and smoking cigarettes if we try surviving without them. Really that is not the case. What we gain is so much more than what we give up. It's not just about preventing something bad from happening, it's about the quality of life. Then it becomes an equation that makes sense - if it's pleasurable, it's sustainable.

THE BIG PICTURE TO HEALTH AND WELLNESS

Study after study has shown that people feel lonely, depressed, and isolated, which I think is the real pandemic besides COVID. People are now 3 to 10 times more likely to get sick and die prematurely. Whereas anything that brings us together is healing. Healing comes from the root "to make it whole." For example, David Spiegel did a study that found that women with metastatic breast cancer that had a support group doubled their survival because they had a safe place where they could connect deeply with other people. These gatherings were once a week for a year.

Also, meditation gives you that experience of what I call "a double vision"- that on one level, we are separate. You are you, and I am me. But on another level, we are all interconnected, and we are all a part of something larger that connects us. The understanding of this kind of intimacy is also healing.

Can I challenge you to move from the "I" of illness to the "we" of wellness?

Aldous Huxley talks about some spiritual truths like the perennial philosophy- altruism, forgiveness, compassion, and love. These free us, as well as others, from our suffering, and to the degree, it brings us closer to people. This is healing.

When I consider the conspiracy of love when someone is suffering, there's an openness to change that you don't always find, because change is hard. If we can meet people when they are suffering and show them how they can use that suffering as a doorway for transforming their lives, it enables us to reclaim our role as healers and not just as technicians.

After 44 years of doing this work, I'm more passionate than ever about doing it. Tech lifestyle medicine is an incredibly rewarding way to practice for both the practitioners, as well as for the patients. It enables us to help people use their suffering as a doorway or catalyst for transforming their lives in ways that go beyond just the physical to the things that matter most.

Chapter Three

David L. Katz MD - Is Lifestyle Medicine the Best Medicine We Have Got?

Dr. Katz is the founding Director of Yale University's Preventive Research Center, Past President of the American College of Lifestyle Medicine, Founder of True Health Initiative, and developer of Diet ID.
↗ davidkatzmd.com

Arguably, in most parts of the world, there are no proper healthcare systems. Rather, we find disease care systems. This means we only wait for things to go badly, then we intervene. However, there are minor exceptions. For example, some of the fundamentals of preventative medicine, cancer screening, and screening for cardio metabolic risk factors, all involve looking for vulnerability before the catastrophe. Most practices are designed to wait for a health crisis.

Nearly 30 years ago I went through my training in internal medicine, and much appreciated the privilege of taking care of people in moments of acute care need. It is a rarefied privilege to be the one to respond "in the moment" of deepest need and gravest anguish, and to be the remedy to this. It is an honor and privilege of being a clinician.

For decades, hospitals have been filling their beds with patient health issues that are avoidable. There are all sorts of ways to prevent this. Rather than trying to unscramble an egg, which doesn't work, we should be looking at preventative measures. Just like the nursery rhyme, Humpty Dumpty. "Humpty Dumpty sat on the wall. Humpty Dumpty had a great fall. All the king's horses and all the king's men couldn't put Humpty together again."

At an early point in my career, I recognized that when spending 110 hours a week in the hospital, we were all playing the part of all the king's men trying to unscramble everyone. We would never succeed; we would never put vitality back together again.

Then to the question, "Is Lifestyle Medicine the Best Medicine We Have Got?" The answer is *"Yes"* because lifestyle medicine can treat acute diseases, as well as chronic issues.

Dr. Dean Ornish, a hero to the world of lifestyle medicine, has shown that lifestyle intervention can do what coronary artery bypass grafts cannot do. In alignment with the Ornish intervention program, the Esselstyn program offers a very similar approach to coronary bypass surgery, which is lifestyle changes. Both systems seek to prevent and reverse heart disease and other chronic health issues.

We have seen that lifestyle changes can offer the same results as Metformin, a drug to address type 2 diabetes in high-risk people. Lifestyle changes offer acute care medicine, disease treatment, disease management, and disease reversal. It is as good as everything medicine has to offer. It is even the better option because it can also cultivate vitality at its origin before any negative health issues even begin. Nothing in medicine can do this except for lifestyle changes. Healthy lifestyle practices are where health and vitality begin.

Biomedicine and how it impacts the planet, is one area of life that some people are concerned about. The planet pays a big price for the destruction from factory waste in producing drugs, and continually exploring new technologies. Thankfully, there is work being done on alternatives to combat climate change and preserve biodiversity around the world.

Lifestyle medicine can improve health and prevent illness without destroying the planet. It alone offers promise to people and the planet alike through:

- Healthy disease management
- Preventative measures
- Lifestyle management practices
- Disease reversal through lifestyle improvements
- Cultivating vitality at the core
- Encouraging exercise, movement, and outdoor activities
- Healthy diet and nutrition

Not only does individual health improve by practicing lifestyle medicine, but the planet does also. Those living the lifestyle of care impact the planet by practicing biodiversity, which brings together humans with nature. There is an innate connection found there. When people care for nature, they care for themselves, and vice versa. This lifestyle also pays-it-forward to future generations. This is the best kind of medicine.

Now, let us talk about science, and talk about it correctly. On one hand, lifestyle results can appear very clear. For example, let's look at the Blue Zones, the geographically areas around the planet where people seem to live the longest. People who get the basic lifestyle medicine formula right, live longer than most. And they prosper with vitality, fulfilling the Vulcan pledge- live long, and prosper.

Blue Zone blessings include longevity, vitality, a good night's sleep, and often an easy transition in death. Let's face it, we are all going to check out at some point. And let's hope it can be peacefully, and not with all kinds of wires and tubes piped into our bodies. That is how it plays out in the Blue Zones. People live to be 100 or more; they stay vital until the very end. Most of these healthy centenarians are known to simply go to bed one night, and

30

not wake up the next day. That is most people's preferred way to transcend.

The times we live in are so fraught and everything can be weaponized. We often point to something that substantiates our point of view and act as if it is the only evidence that matters. We can all benefit from a change in this dogma. It causes a lot of barking with not much listening. And we could all do a better job of listening.

Having conducted and published dozens of randomized control trials, I can rightly say this is not always the best way to come to conclusions. We know a lot of things profoundly well that have never been studied formally. For example, I have raised five children to adulthood. I knew all along, it was a good idea for them not to run with scissors without needing to see a randomized control trial on the topic. I knew too that they really ought to look both ways before crossing a busy street. But again, we have never seen any official science done on this. There is a lot that we know without the scientific studies, research, and reports. A lot of people "want to see the evidence." The evidence is a giant mass of consistent perceptions and experiences.

With lifestyle medicine, what we need to think about is how we can leverage the available science while in the process of more science and study. What science do we have? What science do we need? A few colleagues and I, commissioned by the American College of Lifestyle Medicine, have worked on this very issue. I was privileged to work with giants in the field of evidence related lifestyle, like Walter Willett. Willett is an American physician and nutrition researcher. He was also chair to the Department of Nutrition at the Harvard School of Public Health, between 1991 and 2017.

Together we published a paper in a methodology journal called *HELM, Hierarchies of Evidence applied to Lifestyle*

Medicine. It was argued that the kind of evidence you need must suit the question you're asking. If you are asking, "Will this help people live longer and better?" you can't do a randomized control study. You can't randomly assign people to eat vegan or paleo for 100 years. Nobody is going to play that game. We determined a better way to do this was to combine basic science and mechanistic studies with:

- In-vitro studies
- Observational studies
- Intervention studies.

This method offers a way to pull the information together that is needed, with the evidence, and get a good baseline to begin additional studies with.

One of the often-limiting factors in our lives, whether we like it or not, is money. If we want sustainable interventions in any given system, we need to be prepared to contribute financial support. For example, making the case that when we positively intervene with lifestyle, we are saving both lives and money. This is one of the important frontiers we are currently breaking through. Because of our ability to measure diet quality objectively and effortlessly, my colleagues and I at Diet ID are involved in just this.

We're introducing a Return-On-Investment (ROI) calculator which can help improve diet quality. We use the Healthy Eating Index-2015, in a population with epidemiology resembling most adults in the United States and being ethnocentric. But this could be translated to any group of people. As an example, in a population of 1000 people, like adults in the United States, if you improve diet quality from here to here, how much money would you save? And how fast would you perceive the savings? So, we have designed a calculator where you can plug in any numbers you'd like and generate results. More research and evidence are needed to start convincing people that there is an economic motive as well- to transform a disease care system into the healthcare system we all aspire to have.

Another issue, beyond finances, is the information people are daily inundated with. You hear people say, you can't eat this, or you should eat that. This leaves a tremendous industry in disagreement. The misguided notion that no two nutrition experts agree on anything is completely false.

Everything going on in the world around us is part of lifestyle, and everything impacts all of us. Events and situations that cause anxiety or stress are part of a lifestyle. Political turmoil is part of lifestyle, whether we like it or not. Anything that has us lying awake at night, fretting when we should be relaxing and sleeping, is infiltrating our lifestyle.

I believe that the single greatest plague we face right now is not SARS or Covid; its dissent and discord. We tend to rush into judgment before listening to one another. This is because we often fail to have civil discourse, with a belief that one person has to be right, while the other has to be wrong. Maybe one can be a bit right and another one can also be a bit right. Or maybe if we hybridize our beliefs and respect each other's thoughts and opinions, we'd all get along better. There seems to be a perception that no two nutrition experts agree. This is a false perception.

As an example, if you investigate Dean Ornish's dietary model, you'll see he teaches plant-based diets and low-fat eating. If you look into Frank Hue's practices, the Chair of Nutrition at Harvard, you will learn much about the plant-based, Mediterranean diet.

Both men have spent their careers devoted to and studying two very different dietary models. Did I just call it "Very different?" I did, but it's not really. If you ask the two of them, what are the fundamental principles of a health-promoting diet, their answers would be 95% the same. The 5% is what makes their points of view unique to them. That's what they talk about. We all do that. So, I tested this hypothesis. First, in 2015, I was privileged to co-chair a conference in Boston, with Walter Willett, who was Chair of Nutrition at Harvard at the time. The conference called "Common Ground" was organized by Oldways, a great nonprofit. We brought in opposing nutrition factions from all over the world.

There were experts representing every diet under the sun - Paleo, Mediterranean, vegan, the dairy industry, the beef industry, and others. Our audience was a mixed bag of influencers, dietitians, bloggers, and nutrition journalists. We spent three days presenting to all of them, but the real work was in between the presentations.

We were together in a great big boardroom, and I was the choreographer working toward a consensus statement. We were all out there presenting our view of the world through our own windows. But what was the common denominator? We drafted a consensus statement and published it. We agreed 85 to 90% on a best diet plan with lifestyle practices.

The bedrock of it, Michael Pollan got it down to seven words, **"Eat food, not too much, mostly plants.** So real food, not hyper-processed, glow in the dark, Frankenfood. Real food direct from nature and plants predominant dietary patterns. Get that right and you can't go too far wrong." We published this as a result of the Oldways Common Ground Conference. Michael Pollen has since published a New York Times bestseller, *This is Your Mind on Plants,* available in hard copy and on audible. [13]

---

[13] https://michaelpollan.com/books/this-is-your-mind-on-plants/

34

It would be nice if this could be an ongoing campaign with colleagues from all around the world to agree and say, "We agree about almost everything."

Oldways, the organizer of the conference, is a federally-registered nonprofit, 501C3, with nearly 500 members in the council from 50 or so countries. The group includes the world's leading experts in food and nutrition involved with:

- The Paleo diet
- Leading experts on vegan and vegetarian diets
- Experts in sustainability and biodiversity
- The culinary arts
- The Mediterranean diet
- Latin American and African Heritage health advisory

All these groups come together in agreement to the fundamentals of Lifestyle Medicine, including diet, and agree about what matters most. When brought together with a common cause their practices are shown to eliminate at least 80% of premature death and chronic disease in the modern world. [14]

A most recent book of mine, in fourth edition, is *Nutrition in Clinical Practice*. It's available on Amazon in book and Kindle format. The book is my magnum opus, being the truth about foods. This health professional's guide provides well-informed, compassionate, and effective dietary and weight-management advice. My proceeds from this book are donated to a great cause in support of the True Health Initiative. [15]

Why do I believe I know the truth about foods? And how do I understand the falsehoods that stand between people regarding

---

[14] https://oldwayspt.org/health-studies

[15] https://www.truehealthinitiative.org/news/nutrition-counseling-clinical-practice/

their food beliefs and practices? Because all I have seen and studied has shown me what Michael Pollen's seven words has summed up, "Eat food, not too much, mostly plants." This was the basis of my 200,000 words in *Nutrition in Clinical Practice*. It, however, seems difficult for most people to embrace this simple fundamental truth.

Why did I go to length in explaining this simple principle in my book? How do we know who we can trust? What evidence is there to back it up? Who benefits from this understanding? And who benefits from keeping this simple truth hidden? Who benefits from the never-ending parade of fad diets, books, and programs?

To answers all these questions, there are a lot of industries and individuals who benefit from misinformation.

"What has happened to the human innate ability of knowing what to eat?" This should be the question.

All wild species on the planet know what to eat. Giraffes don't mistakenly eat wildebeest carcasses. They are herbivores; they know what they're supposed to eat.

Similarly, lions might look at the grass and think it looks tasty. No. Because they are obligate carnivores. They do what they must do to survive. Every wild animal on the planet knows what to eat. And when it comes to domestic animals, for the most part, we know what to feed them. For example, I have a horse; I am an equestrian. I have no confusion with what to feed my horse. I don't need genotype to know that my horse eats oats, grass, and hay. He is a horse. It is amazing to me that we humans are so arrogant that we think we are all so special.

Everything else in nature knows what to eat without doing randomized control trials and meta-analyses. But humans, we can't possibly know what to feed ourselves without boatloads of science, and a need to feel special.

36

Do we not hear these statements from people on a regular basis?

- I'm glucose intolerant.
- I can't eat greens; they will interfere with my medications.
- I can't have dairy.
- I'm a vegan.
- I only eat Paleo.
- I'm on a "special" diet.
- I just do keto.
- I'm doing intermittent fasting.
- I'm working with my microbiome type.

Everyone has a need to feel special, and yes, we are each special. But we are all very close cousins. We are all one big family. We are Homo sapiens together. We are one kind of animal more alike than different, and the fundamentals of eating well are of the same basis.

So again, I remind us all, "Eat food, not too much, mostly plants."

This can leave a lot to the imagination, so where do we go from here?

If we eat mostly vegetables, fruits, whole grains, beans, lentils, nuts, and seeds, and when we are thirsty, we mostly drink plain water, then any variant on the theme would probably be okay. You could be pescatarian, flexitarian, vegetarian, vegan, low-fat vegan, or high-fat vegan. You could even manage Paleo. You could follow this simple principle and be low carb with almost any variant you like.

The fundamental theme should not be negotiable. It is not negotiable that my horse eat grass, that lions eat wildebeest, or that elephants eat leaves. And you know, we are a kind of animal. So, remember to eat food, not too much, and mostly plants.

My training in internal medicine began in 1988. I finished medical school in 1991 and immediately started into a second residency in preventative medicine at Yale. I finished up in 1993. During this time period I was introduced to a paper on preventative medicine that was published by the Journal of the American Medical Association. The title of the paper is *Actual causes of death in the United States* and is still available for review online in PubMed files. [16]

If you have a chance to read this article, you'll see that nearly all deaths are preventable, minimally 80%. This could even lead you to believe that everything you thought you know about the causes of death in the United States is wrong.

The paper states also, "Actual causes of death in the **modern** world." "Modern" is important because the epidemiology in the European Union, Canada, Australia, and major parts of Southeast Asia, China, Japan, and the United States, all are comparable. Differences are however found in Bangladesh, the Horn of Africa, and in areas where variances in epidemiology can predicate socioeconomic status levels of development.

From a 2016, Huffpost article by Mike McGinnis and Bill Foege,

> *"... millions of signatures on the world's death certificates are all wrong. Cancer doesn't kill you, heart disease doesn't kill you, diabetes doesn't kill you, what kills you is the antecedent behavior that you have done to cause this pathology that shows up after the fact. The implication of this is immense.*

---

[16] http://pubmed.ncbi.nlm.nih.gov/8411605/

The Medical Industrial Complex pays no attention because it is so busy getting rich providing pills and surgery and devices that it cannot address the ultimate issue which is behavior change. We don't die, we kill ourselves. But there is no pill for behavior change or operation or device. If there is no market it doesn't seem to get done." [17]

McGinnis and Foege are two preeminent epidemiologists with long science careers. Their details of the above statement is that, "what we think is the cause of death is what gets listed on a death certificate." This is usually signed-off on by a sleepy medical resident at three o'clock in the morning.

In fact, what happens is, somebody dies of heart failure after having a heart attack. The cause of death is written as "atherosclerotic", disease of the cardiovascular system. In other words, they died of heart disease.

McGinnis and Foege questioned, "What caused the atherosclerosis in the first place?" They wanted to know the root cause. And with this information is there something that can be done to help further life expectancy in others?

They enumerated a list of ten factors, which collectively accounted for almost every premature death in the United States each year. One incredible thing about their list is that it consisted of just ten issues. Secondly, everything on the list is modifiable today in 2021. The modification includes personal behavior and habits, and exposures to environmental toxins.

Sometimes the best defense of the human body resides with each individual. Sometimes it resides with the body politic. Let's define "body politic" as a collectiveness of an organized group of citizens.

---

[17] https://www.huffpost.com/entry/dare-to-be-100-actual-causes-of-death_b_8991838

Both of these offer opportunities we can take a deep dive into. This is what captured my imagination and changed the course of my entire career. Learning this after being newly minted as a preventive medicine specialist was the game changer.

After reading the paper stating that 80% of premature death and chronic disease is attributable to just three areas, we know are fixable, I knew what my life work needed to focus on.

THREE PROBLEMS	THREE SOLUTIONS
- Tobacco use	- Food
- Poor diet	- Forks
- Lack of exercise	- Fingers

Each of these health issues have impacted everyone's life in one way or another.

- Chronic disease
- Heart disease
- Cancer
- Stroke
- Diabetes
- Dementia

I invite you to think about a day you got some bad news. Think about the deep sadness you felt towards those you love and knew were hurting. And all those affected by a preventable condition. In your gut, feel the emotions if this hadn't happened. This is what the 80% reduction in the burden to chronic disease and premature death would feel like. Feel the promise of a world where eight in ten heart attacks, strokes, diabetes, cancers, and dementia diagnoses or deaths did not occur.

The public has been dupped with fiction. Fiction that leads us to believe that chronic health conditions are normal, and we blindly accept the public health narratives.

Twenty years ago, I set out to help reverse the trends in chronic disease. I set out to be part of the remedy for elevating standards of dietary knowledge around the world. I don't feel that we are winning this war.

The same goes for environmental degradation. It seems that all healthy trends, for man and the planet, continue going in the wrong direction. This is not a time to be complacent.

In terms of health professionals, lifestyle medicine has made some strides. I would love to say we are winning the war, that we are saving the planet, and that we are increasing longevity to all of mankind. But epidemiology is a harsh rebuttal showing us these facts.

- Chronic disease around the world is on the rise.
- Obesity around the world continues to increase.
- Downgrading of diets continue around the world with lower quality foods and higher intakes.
- Negative environmental impacts continue to increase the toxins in our air, food, water, and soil.

For any real solutions, we need to be brutally honest about the tough fight this is. Lifestyle medicine is inspiring me, and I hope you also.

I am privileged to be a past president of the American College of Lifestyle Medicine. I attend and often speak at the meetings and conferences. My participation has brought me to all 50 states as well as six continents. No other conferences I've been to have had the high energy as the Lifestyle Medicine Conferences. It's always an exciting and incredible experience. I believe the reason is due to the offering of "hope."

Hope is offered, for a better way of life, and for a deeper calling. People are encouraged with the hope of being able to offer additional years of life, to others and themselves. And for doing it in a way that is kind and gentle to their fellow creatures. It's always very inspiring. When we learn to be part of the solutions, we increase our faith in a different way for the future. I always come away full of hope.

The Book of Hope, by Jane Goodall, is a recent addition to my library. Who better than Goodall to be the ambassador of hope after all the positive changes she's made in the world? Lifestyle Medicine should be as inspiring as she is.

There are many ways that people can be engaged in changing the world, especially with living in the digital age. Are there ways you can incorporate the practice and teachings of Lifestyle Medicine into your life? There are many models for this that we can look at.

1) Telemedicine- Seeing patients remotely as you incorporate Lifestyle Medicine into your current practice.
   - Tremendously popular since the pandemic
   - Reimbursable in most cases
   - Offers wide audience potential
2) Become an expert in Lifestyle Medicine and offer health coaching.
   - New ways of offering structuring care through group visits and programs.
     - The dialogue could look something like this:

       "I can't tell you very much about diet in 10 minutes or even 15. I need an hour and a half. But there is no way I can take care of you for an hour and a half, and bill you what I need to bill you without you never coming back. If I don't bill you enough, I don't make money, and I go out of business. So, what do we do? Well, we have a group visit of 12 or 15 people all at the same time. And instead of everybody getting eight minutes, everybody gets 90, everybody gets billed, and I am fully paid for the hour and a half."

- Emphasis that group programs build a sense of community.
- This is a very simple yet powerful model.

3) Lifestyle Medicine offers a host of entrepreneurial opportunities.
    - In my case, I developed Diet ID. This is a cutting-edge, health tool for accessing and promoting good dietary habits. This technology is used by healthcare practitioners, health coaches, and researchers.

The question then becomes what now?

If you're practicing any type of medicine or health coaching, you can simply jump right in. If you're part of team, you can refer colleagues to the Lifestyle Medicine program. If you are neither of these, you can look at digital and social networking to share information about it.

Not everybody needs to know everything, but everybody can participate in some way to making changes to the new way of healthcare.

Even for those who don't want to be experts in Lifestyle Medicine, you can connect with those who are and help them take better care of their patients and even themselves.

Incorporating Lifestyle Medicine into your life is the antidote to burnout!

Chapter Four

T. Colin Campbell Ph.D. - Nutrition Reformation and Renaissance (The China Study)

T. Colin Campbell, Ph.D., is a Jacob Gould Schurman Professor Emeritus of Nutritional Biochemistry at Cornell University, Project Director of the acclaimed China-Oxford-Cornell Diet and Health Project, coauthor of The China Study, and author of Whole: Rethinking the Science of Nutrition.
↗ nutritionstudies.org

Lifestyle medicine is going to be the future of medicine. And as far as lifestyle is concerned, we should stop and think for a moment. What does that mean? It means getting good sleep, an adequate amount of sunshine, and probably a matter of relaxation and physical activity. The one perspective on lifestyle medicine, or the one that has the most far-reaching effect is food choice. By food choice, we are talking about the impact of food on human, planetary, and environmental health.

Let us have a look first at the current system that we're living with to get a better fixation on what lifestyle medicine might mean.

Let's look at some data on the United States that is most familiar with us, and because the US tends to be a premier Western medicine type of society. The current system, referred to as Western medicine, denotes the following:

- Per capita cost of healthcare (#1)
- Per capita cost of pharmaceuticals (#1)
- Declining life expectancy (#26)
- Per capita cost of healthcare (#1)
- Obesity (#3)

- Prescription drug side effects as cause of death (#4 of 10 in US)

This is data from the Office of Economic Cooperation Development comparing the United States with 35 mostly European, and a few Asian countries. Here in the United States, we are number one in the per capita cost of health care. We also are number one in the use and the cost of pharmaceuticals, but even with that, during the last four to five years, we've seen declining life expectancy.

Presently, we're ranked somewhere around number 26 out of 35 in these Western medicine-type countries. We're number three in prevalence of obesity, and then number one in our per capita cost of pharmaceuticals. And lest we not forget the cost of this being more than just financial; but the side effects of pharmaceuticals, including death. The side effects from the use of pharmaceutical drugs rank number 4 among the 10 leading causes of death in the US.

So, we use a lot of drugs, and we pay a big cost. This system leads to an unequal health care problem. Among the Western countries, the United States experiences high health care costs and low health returns. Good for business, but bad for health.

Let's look next at the environment, which of course involves both the USA and obviously, all countries in the world. There are many identifiable problems:

- Climate warming
- Ocean pollution
- Aquifer water lowering
- Topsoil loss
- Deforestation, especially in tropical and subtropical areas of the world
- A mass extinction of all species

45

All of these are, fair to say, basically at present, uncontrolled. This tells us an environmental catastrophe is coming. Writers and researchers in this field with the best data are suggesting that close to 90% of the human race will be lost by the end of the century. This gives us some perspective because we're talking about our grandchildren. We must start taking this seriously.

Think about these two sets of problems. One, the personal health equation, and the other has to do with environmental health. Do both areas have an independent cause? Or is there a common cause? Of course, they have their characteristics and how they work on each problem. But is there an overhanging sky for both? Is there a common solution there?

As far as a common cause and a common solution is concerned, with health and environmental issues, here is a hint. An essentially significant amount of research from experts over decades report 85% of chronic disease risk and the cost associated with it has a direct relationship to diet. In turn, if it is due to diet, I offer a hypothesis concerning the practice of a plant-based, protein diet; that the dietary factor most predictive of chronic disease is simply choosing to consume animal protein. That being said, what data do we have concerning animal protein and chronic disease?

Here are a series of screenshots from researchers in earlier times that I find very intriguing. These screenshots are simply graphs representing the emergence of specific diseases relative to diet.

46

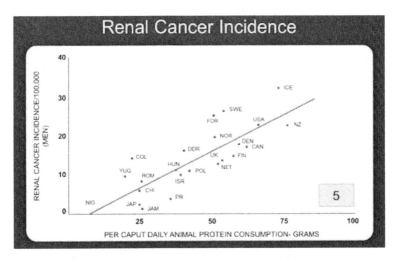

In this case, these are kidney cancer incidents, relative to the consumption of animal protein. Notice the rather straight downward projection, right to left.

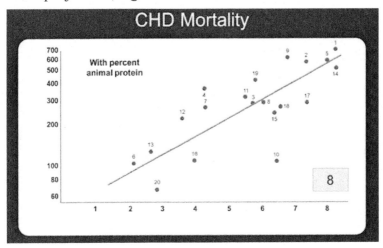

This shows coronary heart disease (CHD) related to consumption of animal protein, in different countries. This particular information was published in 1959. Notice the similar projection.

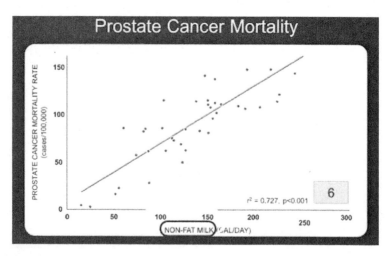

The above chart provides statistics for prostate cancer, and the consumption of non-fat milk. Non-fat milk related to prostate cancer mortality shows a straight linear regression (from right to left).

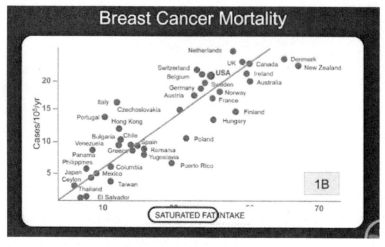

This chart shows the relationship between saturated fat consumption and breast cancer. Again, we see a line almost the same as the others.

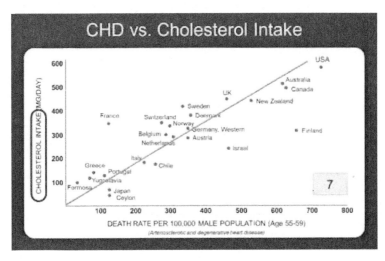

Here is the death rate for heart disease from the consumption of cholesterol.

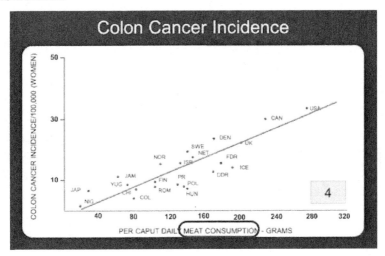

This shows us the relationship between colon cancer and meat consumption.

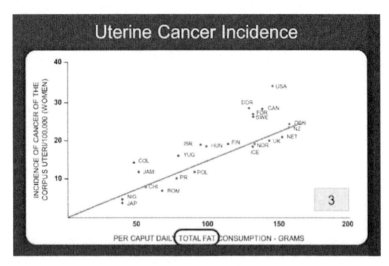

And lastly, here is one for urine cancer and total fat consumption.

What can we say about these seven screenshots? These screenshots present as researchers have shown them. I superimposed the linear line using the same metric.

What we see with these lines is that the line goes down and intercepts near the X Y origin. So, in theory, what it suggests is, any introduction of these substances was associated with a possible increased risk for these diseases. Non-fat milk, saturated fat, cholesterol, meat, and total fat, are not to be seen separately. They are markers of animal protein-based foods.

In contrast, when one of the researchers on the breast cancer story published his work on animal protein, he also found that plant protein didn't have the same type of relationship. I want to make this point. These regression lines that we have seen, show an increase in animal protein consumption from animal protein foods, versus the outcome of various diseases.

In summary, increased intake of dietary animal protein increases the risk for multiple diseases. This goes along with the idea that an increase of dietary animal foods- meat, milk, and eggs, combines with, quite naturally, a decreased intake of plant foods like vegetables, fruits, grains, and seeds, all of which tend to decrease disease risk. So those correlational notes, regression lines you saw in the screenshots, for example, represent a relationship with these animal-protein intakes.

It stands to reason than that intake of animal protein foods would cause a decreased intake of plant foods. Plant foods, of course, have very good antioxidants, very good nutrients, and their complex carbohydrates have proven dietary fiber, as well as the right kind of protein. Animal foods don't have these.

My next questions then become, "How can we explain the relationship between these disease associations with animal protein?" "What's the mechanism?"

I am taking you to some evidence from the laboratory, in this case, evidence from my laboratory, showing how I got caught up in this story. This goes back a few years and shows a study from India on experimental animals that were administered a carcinogen to cause liver cancer. These administrators thought that if they gave more dietary protein, 20% as opposed to 5%, they would be able to repress the formation of cancer.

It turned out that the animals that were given the 20% protein, considered to be good levels versus regular levels, got cancer. The ones that were given 5% protein did not. Exactly the opposite of what they thought happened. They didn't believe their data.

This correlates with a Philippine program I was responsible for involving malnourished children. My work in the Philippines was to develop a model for malnourished children principally by increasing their consumption of protein, ideally animal protein.

The studies were alarming because they both suggested that more protein, means more cancer. I came back home and started my research career. Nearly fifty years have passed since.

More recent data, from 1992, caught my attention.

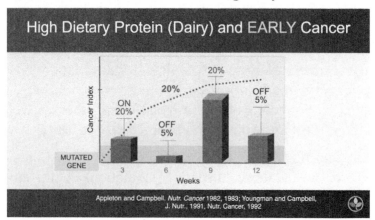

This shows the emergence of cancer in an experimental animal model. The emergence of cancer, specifically liver cancer, over 12 weeks, started with a mutated gene. There are two different levels of protein, as in the Indian study. First is the dairy protein. When dairy protein is fed at 20% of calories, we see cancer growing rather well, but at 5%, there was none. This also was in alignment with what I saw among the starving and malnourished Philippine children.

I had some students who were involved in this study with me, but we did something that was rather stark. What we learned was that if we switched the diet from 20% to 5%, back then 20%, then again back to 5%, we could turn cancer on and off. Turning it on and off; this was eye-popping. That kind of set- 20-5-20-5, giving higher levels of animal protein turned on cancer cells, while reducing, turned off the cells. This also suggested something else that was very provocative at the time. Nutrition rather than genes, mutation if you will, primarily controls cancer development.

The next question I had was, "Okay, is this true?"

I found this somewhat hard to believe because I was raised on a dairy farm. I also did my graduate work of my doctoral dissertation on promoting the consumption of animal protein. So, I was very pinned to ask these questions:

- What is the mechanism?
- Is it the protein effect?
- Why should we want to know the biochemical mechanism?

Well, it helps us to understand and get some confirmation of what we saw. But the other possibility was, if we can understand this specific mechanism, maybe we can develop a drug to block this protein effect. That was the thinking back in the day. And so, I'm going to share with you a quick summary of what we learned over the next ten to twelve years asking these questions.

Here is a scheme that we tend to use in cancer research.

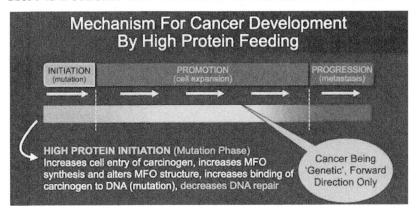

There are three phases.

- Phase 1- The initiation phase when mutations are forming.
- Phase 2- Promotion, when the cells accumulate in the body.

53

- Phase 3- Progression of the cells getting nasty and possibly metastasizing to other tissues.

What we found from Phase 1 was very interesting. The high protein diet increased the rate of the entry of the carcinogen into the cell, and also increased an enzyme referred to as mixed-function oxidase. This is an increase in an enzyme that metabolizes the carcinogen to produce a very active product. This product binds the DNA. We found that the high protein diet increased the amount of this particular enzyme and also altered its structure in such a way that it was more active. We learned that a high animal protein diet increased the amount of the carcinogen and bonded it to the DNA, which is the source of mutation. That is how the mutation starts and that is how cancer begins.

Then we learned something else very interesting. We have in our systems the natural ability to repair all those DNA damages that occur from time to time. A high protein diet compromises and represses the one mechanism that we have to protect ourselves.

The high animal protein diet is slow to increase the mechanisms that keep the body healthy, while fast to increase the damaging mechanisms. I couldn't tell which one was the key mechanism. This is yet to be determined.

Going to the second stage of promotion, you'll notice here the double, reversible arrows as opposed to the person.

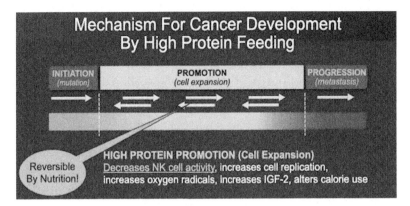

The double arrows are something I mentioned earlier where we can turn cancer on and off. So, we looked for mechanisms there, and we found a bunch again.

First of all, the high protein animal diet decreased another one of these protective mechanisms, which is the production of so-called "natural killer cells", a product of the immune system. A decrease in natural killer cells, therefore, allows cancer to grow and increases the rate at which cancer cells are dividing. It increased the oxygen free radical which promotes cancer, increased a hormone, and so forth and so on.

There are a multitude of mechanisms and here is the summary. We looked for each of these and found eight mechanisms. Of these eight, we found that animal protein increased the mechanisms that cause cancer and are damaging while at the same time decreasing the two mechanisms that protects us.

In other words, a chain of 10 for 10 was changed by high protein diets. And fascinatingly, all tens were working in synchrony; this was amazing. This for me raised a red flag for creating drugs which have side effects. Drugs could be developed and used by any one of these mechanisms. If we can determine the mechanism for a better effect, then we can find a chemical, a drug essentially, to block it.

With drugs presenting side effects, what are we going to do with something like this? Are we going to make a drug for each of these ten mechanisms, dozens, or maybe hundreds more mechanisms that we don't even know about? Would a better idea be to shave the amount of protein intake and work synchronistical and naturally with our bodies?

This raises questions about our insatiable demand for animal protein which has almost no limits historically, scholarly, socially, politically, or economically. We should question the role of animal protein as a so-called "high-quality protein", which it is not. These questions could also be very damaging for one's career, to say the least. It defines the Western medical system and our consumption of animal protein. So much for the animal protein part of my little story.

Here is a second part. This applies directly to lifestyle medicine. It's a second perspective that has to do with the way nutrition works, or nutrients work. I will share with you a study that came out first in the early 1980s, just about the time we were doing our work. It has to do with lung cancer and what they learned in the studies amongst heavy smokers- those smoking for more than 30 years. What they learned was that the smokers consuming or having the highest level of beta carotene (vitamin A from plants) in their blood had the least cancer. There was a remarkable dose-response relationship.

This caused researchers to get interested in an idea. Let's take the beta carotene out of foods and put it into pills. Maybe we can prevent lung cancer in smokers? A study was then undertaken among 29,000 male smokers. It was a joint study between Norwegian and American researchers at the time. They intended for the study to last for eight years, but they had to cut it short after five because of the following reasons:

- The smokers who were consuming beta carotene ended up seeing a decrease in lung cancer risk and it was statistically significant.
- There was a decrease of almost 20% in just the first five years among cancer rates.
- In contrast, the ones who were given the beta-carotene supplement, increased lung cancer again by almost 20%.
- The opposite of what was expected.

Here is a nutrient, a very important nutrient. When it comes from food, it does a good job but when it is taken out and made into a supplement, it has the opposite effect.

"Wholelism" to me, is lifestyle medicine – nutrition working through food. All nutrition works together to create a response. Supplements, in contrast, are more of western medicine philosophy where we tend to do one thing at a time via drugs. That's what we call "reductionism", and that's the central theme of Western medicine.

This gives me a definition of nutrition. Nutrition, for me, is holistic and involves multiple nutrients. I'm talking about hundreds of thousands, even far more possibly natural chemicals and foods that work together to create a response. I'm talking about multiple mechanisms for each nutrient.

Imagine this, countless nutrients, each one having countless mechanisms to bruise a whole array of diseases. If we address a broad range of health issues, the results would be multiple health improvements.

The biology of the system is extraordinarily complex when we look at all the parts. There are almost an infinite number of factors, nutrients, and diseases that we could talk about, and this can be very confusing. But in contrast, nutrition alone or just eating the right foods can do it all at the same time.

I have two suggestions.

1) Consume whole foods for a healthy nutritional foundation.
2) Focus on consuming whole plants.

Lifestyle Medicine is easy. Less support from medicine with a balance of nutrition and food consumption equates to good health. Keeping it simple, we recommend consuming plants, not animals. In this way we consume nutrients in their wholistic and most natural form.

Here in a nutshell is lifestyle medicine in contrast to reductions. One disease, one cause, and one mechanism, that is the heart and soul of Western medicine. It is a huge enterprise. Their products are said to be targeted, and this sound great. But do we make a specific chemical to target a specific mechanism even when there is no real specific mechanism? That is why we have all the side effects and such a cornucopia of drugs, all working together, or really "not" working so well together. This explains why side effects are so common. A "Wholelist" nutritional approach, in contrast, works everything together without side effects. This is the reason "wholistic nutrition" is not taught at reductionist medical schools. The two are opposites. And therefore, why nutrition is not considered a medical science.

This is also why in experimental nutritional research we tend to focus on individual interactions. Like focusing on individual drugs, we focus on individual interests. This is a source of enormous confusion. Here's where the confusion comes for the public at large. When we hear of a new discovery of a nutrient or nutrient-like substance, it ends up involving one more disease. Always one more mechanism to impress us. This is Western medicine in a nutshell. The focus is about working on separate parts, and not the whole. Therein lies the problem.

Nutrition deals with the whole. Western medicine deals with thousands of different kinds of drugs for specific issues. The main solution for a healthy lifestyle is, eat the right food.

The studies mentioned herein are discussed extensively in the books I've written. My first is *The China Study*. It was published in 2005 and republished in 2016. This book has been translated into fifty foreign languages. What a wonderful surprise to me that the world showed so much interest.

My second book is *Whole: Rethinking the Science of Nutrition*, a New York Times bestseller and best for describing the concept of Wholeism.

My most current work is *The Future of Nutrition: An Insider's Look at the Science, Why We Keep Getting It Wrong, and How to Start Getting It Right*.

I enjoy sharing and talking about nutrition, and a future that takes into consideration all I have learned and shared. This future focuses on using food to solve our health problems instead of relying on chemicals every time we have any type of health issue.

Chapter Five

Bruce Lipton Ph.D. - Medicine, Consciousness, and Healing

Bruce Lipton is the bestselling author of The Biology of Belief, former research scientist, medical school professor, and an internationally recognized leader in Epigenetics and "bridging science and spirit."
↗ brucelipton.com

Healthcare is a big issue. That's because it's almost a global crisis. The amount of money that goes into health care and the outcomes don't match very well. So, there's a global solution and that's what I hope we get a chance to understand.

I was teaching at a medical school years ago and in the first year I taught about cells, cell biology, histology, and embryology, all giving a foundation of how science works. At that time there was an insight called genetic determinism. It was the belief that genes determine the character of your life. How significant could that be? First of all, as far as we knew, we didn't pick the genes we came with. Number two is, if you don't like the characteristic, you can't change the genes you came with. Number three, which is the killer, we were also told that genes turn on and off by themselves. Putting this all together, it means we are victims of our heredity. Whatever is running in your family- cancer, diabetes, Alzheimer's, oh, you have a gene for that. I'm sorry, you're already a victim. You're a victim because the genes are going to turn on and off. They're going to control your life and we have some pharmaceutical drugs for you. This is what I was teaching.

In the laboratory, I was cloning stem cells, and this was over 50 years ago. And yeah, that's a long time, half a century if you say it that way. But over 50 years ago, why was this relevant? It was only a small population in the whole world that even knew what the heck a stem cell was at the time, and I happened to be in the right place at the right time cloning them. And what does all this mean?

I put one stem cell in a dish by itself, it divided every ten or twelve hours versus one, two, and four, eight, sixteen, doublings. After a week, there are 30,000 cells in the Petri dish.

I have 30,000 genetically identical cells. Next, I split them into three different dishes with 10,000 cells in each dish. All dishes are genetically identical cells. But what I did was change the chemical composition of the growth medium. And this is going to come back real big in a minute. I changed the chemical composition of the growth medium which is what we grow cells in and saw that I had three different versions. This is the environment that the cells live in. I have three environments for the three genetically identical cells.

But what happened was, the cells in environment "A" formed muscle; the cells in environment "B" formed bones; and the cells in environment "C" formed fat cells. But what controls the fate of the cells though they were all genetically the same? The only different thing was the environment. And it was like, "Oh my god." This is completely different than the story of genes turning off and on by themselves. This is the environment that regulates the genes. As I started to follow all of this, of course, my colleagues thought I was crazy because everybody was into genes and I was saying, "No, it's not the genes."

This is the foundation of the science that we refer to today as epigenetics. When I say this character is under genetic control, I am saying that the genes control the character. But now I say this character is under epigenetic control. It sounds the same but is revolutionary. Why? "Epi" means above. What do we call skin?

Epidermis, meaning above the dermis. When I ask, "What is epigenetics?" It is "Control" - "epi" - above the genes.

What do I mean? Am I saying the genes controlling us aren't turning on and off? No, it was the environment that is controlling the genes. This is a radical change because if the genes control life, we have no control, we are a victim. But if the environment controls genes, then we can be a master because we can control our environment. And all of a sudden it shows us:

- Genetics, genetic determinism – victim
- Epigenetics - master of your life

Wait, how do the cells in the plastic dish relate to the human body? Good question and here's the good answer. We are skin-covered Petri dishes. Underneath our skin is 50 trillion cells and they have a culture medium. What is a culture medium? A culture medium is the laboratory version of blood. If I grow human cells in a culture dish, I look at what human blood has in it and make a culture medium based on that chemistry. If I grow mouse cells, I look at what mouse blood has in it, etc.

Let us experiment. Culture medium controls the fate of the cells in the plastic dish. But we are skin-covered Petri dishes with 50 trillion cells inside and the original culture medium, blood. It doesn't make a difference if the cell is in a plastic dish, or the cell is in the skin-covered dish; it's still controlled by the environment. It's the chemistry. The culture medium controls my genetics. And then suddenly, this big question comes up, "Who's the chemist?"

Who's making the chemicals that I have inside my blood? The brain is the chemist. It adds these factors to the blood. Now comes the sweet part; what chemistry should be put into the blood? And the answer is, whatever picture you hold in your mind, the brain's job is to translate that picture into complimentary chemistry. If you're visualizing love, the brain will interpret love by putting wonderful chemistry into your blood like dopamine for pleasure, oxytocin for bonding, and growth hormone (when you're in love, you release growth hormone). It enhances your growth and that is why when people fall in love, they glow and are healthy. That's not a coincidence or an accident. That's chemistry. It's chemistry from taking a picture of love and converting it into complimentary chemistry. What if I have a picture of fear? That is different chemistry. In a picture of fear, the brain translates fear into stress hormones and cytokines which influence the immune system, histamine, and things like this are released. Well, that's different chemistry. Love gives us growth, and fear puts us into protection. These are two different states of being.

Ninety percent of doctor visits today are due to people living under stress.

Living in today's world there is a barrage of stressors. Do I have enough money for the rent? Am I going to be able to get food? Am I going to get health care? Can I get money? Will I be living on the street?

Why is stress so critical? The answer, it releases stress hormones. Why do we have a stress response? Let us say, a saber-toothed tiger is coming! We go, "Whoa", and into panic mode. We go from growth into protection. How? Because when we see that tiger, the stress hormones coming from the brain change our biology to "run!" So, we run away from that stress. It takes energy to run away from stress. The body is using energy for a lot of things. If you're just sitting around somewhere, your body energy is in your gut, mainly the viscera. Why? For maintenance of the body, growth of the body, care of the body, and that's what the function of all these organs are. But if you're being chased by a saber-toothed tiger, the blood carries energy. Do I want the energy to be growing in my body? No! I want all the energy to run and fight or flight from that tiger.

When the stress hormones are released into the body, they cause the blood vessels in the gut to squeeze shut because it pushes the blood, which is the energy, to the arms and legs. If I squeeze these blood vessels in what is now the arms or legs, I need to run. I need all that energy. When you're under stress, you shut down growth, maintenance, and taking care of the system because the energy of the system is like, "you don't have to worry about taking care of yourself if that tiger catches you." The first thing that happens is this- you shut down your growth mechanism. Then here comes another one, the immune system. The immune system protects us from internal threats of bacterial and viral infections. The immune system uses a lot of energy. If you've ever been sick, you may not have had the energy to get out of bed, and that's how much energy the immune system uses.

Now, a saber-toothed tiger is chasing me, and I have a bacterial infection. Where do I want to put the energy? The heck with the bacteria! If the tiger catches me, the bacteria are his problem, not mine. We don't want the immune system to be functioning when we're in fight or flight because it takes away too much energy. In this case, stress hormones shut off the immune system. It's so effective that when doctors want to do a transplant of an organ from person A into person B, they don't want person B's immune system to reject the foreign graft. So, they give that patient stress hormones before they do the graft as it inhibits the immune system so that the graft will not be attacked.

There are three effects of stress hormones.

1) Shutting down growth and maintenance.
2) Shutting down the immune system because the energy is needed to run away.
3) It adds insult to the injury we already are facing.

When we're conscious, we're using the forebrain which is creative thinking. When we're under stress, we go to the hindbrain. This is where the reflex-reaction is extremely fast while consciousness is slow. You're in an emergency; it's not time to think, it's time to react. The stress hormones shut off the blood vessels in the gut. They squeeze the blood vessels in the forebrain shut so that the blood with the energy gets pushed to the hindbrain where the reaction is going to occur, and we become less intelligent and more reactionary.

When the system was designed, the only thing we had to run away from was a saber-toothed tiger. After 10 to 15 minutes, if we can get away from the tiger and there is no more threat, the stress system stops, and you go back into growth again. But in today's world, stress is 24/7, 365 days a year.

Human biology was not designed for prolonged chronic stress. The result of this is the health crisis that we're facing today because up to 90% of doctor visits are stress-related ailments. If you want to help people, the first thing is to help and encourage them to get rid of stress. Look at today's world. There are more stressors out there than ever. People turn on the news; hey, everything today was beautiful, but that's not the news. Everything today is scary- you got no money, you got no health care going, all kinds of problems, supply chain shortage, and the list of fears goes on and on. Go to the store, maybe there's nothing there. But the only way out of this problem is not to give people drugs, not to give them vaccinations. The way out of this problem is to have people get healthy. When you hear the news about COVID- we have the vaccine and we have masks, we have social distancing, and then somewhere down the line, they say to get healthy. Are you kidding me? Getting healthy is number one because a healthy immune system will protect you from this and other viruses. Up to 90% of people with COVID infections, didn't even go to a doctor or hospital because their immune system was working okay.

The number one group of people who suffer from COVID, is the aged and infirmed, because their immune systems are already compromised. They're on their last legs. The second group are people with what are called comorbidities, and these are the ones who will experience serious problems with COVID. For people that don't have comorbidities, it's flu but not happy flu, but it will go away in a week or ten days, and you'll be immunized for life.

The problem is that comorbidities are contributing to the serious ailments that people have, like obesity, very high-stress levels, cardiac issues, and organ complications; these are all serious health problems. We can service and survive these health issues, but if you ignore them, then you are ripe for a problem because the first thing is, the stress hormone shuts off your immune system. You are then automatically in a very desperate situation.

What we need to do is change the understanding of health care. I will give this statistic, not out of joy, but out of necessity. In the year 2000, Barbara Starfield published an article in the Journal of the American Medical Association, JAMA. She said, "Medicine in the United States is the third leading cause of death behind cancer and heart disease." Medicine? Yes, it's called iatrogenic illness. A patient goes in for treatment for problem A, the treatment causes problem B, and they die from B. They didn't die from A, they died from the treatment.

That was in 2000. The British Medical Journal recently repeated the same research in 2016, with the same result - medicine is the third leading cause of death in the United States. We pay the most money and have the worst health care. So where is all this money going? We have been led to believe the pharmaceutical company is our friend and that they are here to help us.

First of all, understand the nature of "what is a corporation?" A corporation is a business with the first principle of making a profit for the shareholders.

We think that the number one mission of the pharmaceutical companies is to help us, but their number one mission is for them to make money. This is all legitimate. If a corporation isn't out to try to make more money, then the shareholders can cause the whole thing to collapse. I taught in medical schools, I researched at Stanford Medical School, I am very familiar with the fact that the pharmaceutical companies have their hands in every aspect of medical education. They sell a product. So?

What if I give you health care information to show that you don't have to buy a pharmaceutical agent? That's not what they want to pay for. The idea is, they fund doctors, and they fund medical schools. They fund because outside of the military-industrial complex, they are the second-largest money-making industry in the world. But we can heal without pharmaceuticals. If a pharmaceutical agent can help you, that implies that the chemical you just took matches a receptor in the body that will read that chemical. There must be receptors but why do you think they're there? Waiting for the pharmaceutical company to develop drugs?

No! It was always there. Any receptor in your body that responds to the pharmaceutical agent is also a receptor that responds to a natural agent. That's why the body has the receptor. Your body makes all the drugs that the pharmaceutical companies are selling you. Because if that receptor is in there, it wasn't waiting for the pharmaceutical company to come up with a drug. It was there because we already have it.

67

We have been programmed to believe that we are victims of our heredity. If you believe you're a victim, you also believe there's a rescuer. "I'm a victim, who can help me?" All of a sudden, the pharmaceutical companies come – "we can help you frail human beings." But we're not frail. How come I'm not making the chemistry I need? Well, who's making the chemistry? Oh, the brain. What chemistry? To complement the picture. But what's the picture? Watch the news. You want to see the picture every day, it's very stress-provoking. And again, that's why 90% of doctor visits are directly related to stress.

The brain is taking the picture from the mind and making that into the chemistry that complements that picture. If it's a healthy picture of love, then the chemistry that comes out gives health and vitality. But if it's a picture of fear or stress, like "I'm not going to survive" or whatever it is, that chemistry puts you in protection and that shuts down your growth, your immune system, and the ability to heal yourself shuts down. But a lot of people are out there saying, "Yeah, I have all these positive thoughts, yet, I still have problems."

The exact source of that problem is that the mind is creating the chemistry that controls your genetics and your behavior. There are two minds. One is called the conscious mind and the original mind is called the subconscious mind. The conscious mind is the advanced mind that is based on creativity - creation. That's why we can create things. We always have these imaginations that we can create things. The subconscious mind is a different system. That's the equivalent of a hard drive in a computer. The brain is a computer. It has the same components that a silicon computer has, even though it's a carbon computer.

Imagine you buy a brand-new computer, bring it home, start it, it boots up, the screen lights up, and you try to do something- a spreadsheet, a drawing, something. Then you say, "No, I can't do it." Why? First, you must put programs in the computer before you can use it. This is similar to a child's brain booting-up in the last trimester of pregnancy. But to be functional, it has to have programs. Where do the programs come from? For the first seven years of a child's life, the brain activity is like an EEG - electroencephalograph wires on a person's head. The brain activity of a child for the first seven years is not at the higher vibration of consciousness. It's just below consciousness. The child doesn't even have predominant conscious activity until after age seven.

What's below consciousness? Theta. That's the zone of vibration. What does that represent? Well, it represents imagination. That's how kids have a tea party. They put nothing into the cup, drink nothing from the cup, and yet that was the most wonderful tea they ever had in their life. That's theta. Riding a broom and thinking it's a horse. The mother might say, "Give me the broom." The child is not seeing a broom. The kid is on a horse! Theta - imagination. But here comes the serious part.

Theta is hypnosis. What's the relevance? How many things must a child learn to become a functional member of a family in a community? How many rules? Thousands of rules! Are you going to give this infant a book to read? That is not going to work. You can't give them a lecture. How does a child get to learn thousands of rules? The answer is theta, hypnosis. All they do is watch the mother or father, the siblings, and their community. They watch their behavior in a state of hypnosis. They download the behavior.

So whatever behavior your father was showing, you copy that, if you weren't conscious, you didn't filter it. You didn't say, "Oh, that was a bad thing or a good thing." You weren't even conscious; you were just recording. And it turns out about 70% of the recordings are disempowering or self-sabotaging beliefs. The subconscious programs are put in through age seven. After age seven you have an opportunity to use the conscious mind to create your life.

Now here comes a big problem, the conscious mind can think. For a moment, consider the body as a vehicle with a steering wheel and the conscious mind is driving. Where's it going? The conscious mind is creative. It's going to drive you to its wishes and desires- health, happiness, a great job, love, and joy. That's what the conscious mind is looking for.

The conscious mind can think, but thinking is not looking out but rather looking in. The conscious mind, when it's thinking, stops looking out at the world and thought is inside. But what if I'm driving down the street and suddenly have a thought, and the conscious mind at this point is not driving? Oh my God, no!

Don't worry. Driving is a habit, you learn how to do it, and it automatically means it's a subconscious program. The subconscious mind is an auto pilot. When you are thinking and not looking out at the world, but you're looking in, the subconscious programs take over your life.

Where did they come from? They come from other people, not from you. When you're thinking you're not playing your wishes and desires, or what you want, recognize you are playing programs you've downloaded from other people. I'm going to give you a surprising statistic- 95% of our day is not coming from the creative conscious mind. This 95% of our data is coming from subconscious autopilot programs.

We're not living our lives; we're living the programs that we got from other people. The vast majority of these are disempowering and self-sabotaging beliefs. You might be saying, "Well, if I am sabotaging myself, I would see it!" No, you wouldn't, because when you're thinking, you're not looking out, you're looking in. You don't see the behavior that you're playing out.

I have told a very fundamentally yet profound story for 30 years. You have a friend, and you know your friend's behavior. You also know your friend's parents and one day you see that your friend has the same behavior as their parents. And you want to tell your friend, "Hey, Bill, you're just like your dad." Back away from Bill. The moment you say this, I know what Bill is going to say. He's going to say, "How can you compare me to my dad? I'm nothing like my dad."

Everyone else can see that Bill behaves like his dad. Who's the one that can't see it? Bill! He is not consciously playing his dad's behavior, but the program is, and he's not paying attention. That's the problem.

You play the subconscious programs; you don't even see them. And if they're negative, you will be sabotaging yourself all day playing programs that you don't even see. Imagine we wake up and say, "Today's the day I'm going to find love, today's that day I'm going to get healthy." Good! Eight o'clock in the morning. Let's go. You come home at five o'clock. You didn't find love. You didn't get any healthier. Crappy day. What is the person's thought at that moment? At five o'clock they come home and realize their wishes and desires for that day didn't happen. They think, "I'm a victim. I want to be successful. I want to be healthy. It's those people and that thing, whatever it is, that is making me not healthy. I'm a victim and that means I'm powerless." This is the biggest problem in the entire world.

We are creators of our life, and we are profoundly powerful. Quantum physics is the most valid science on this planet. No science has been studied more or affirmed to be truer than quantum physics. Principle number one in quantum physics says consciousness is creating your life experiences.

Founding father of quantum physics, Max Planck, stated that **"The mind is the matrix of all matter."** What did he mean by this? He meant that the mind is the environment that creates all matters. But if you're playing your programs, you're not creating; your programs are creating.

For 400 years the Jesuits have told their followers, "Give me a child until he is seven and I will show you the man." What did they know? Seven years is programming and 95% of that person's life is coming from the program. If I can program you, I own the character of your life. That's been known for at least 400 years. If you think this isn't being used today, you're not paying attention. An example of modern-day programming is seeing an infant who can hardly walk yet they are carrying around an iPad. That's programming.

Do you see how we are creating our lives? We believe we are victims, and the truth of quantum physics and epigenetics is the biology behind quantum physics. This is the mechanism that shows how consciousness is manifesting our genetics and our behavior. Quantum physics and epigenetics come together and say to us, **"You have to wake up because you're creating. And if you don't like the creation, you have got to change this or that, not the world. Change this or that, and the world will change for you."**

Science is pretty clear on this, yet it seems it's not been integrated into the majority of our beliefs and perspectives.

In health care, aspects of Lifestyle Medicine are- lifestyle, diet, exercise, stress management, social support, and mediation. We know it works, but an underused aspect is a psychosocial stress. Our environment has an impact and it's designed by us as an interaction between the two. A lot of people are constantly wondering, "Why doesn't this work for me then?" The fact is, the human brain, like a computer, must be programmed before you can use it. The programming occurs in the first seven years. What are your programs? You might reply, "I'm thinking I have this belief." Then I would say, "You were programmed before you were born. During the last trimester of pregnancy, you were downloading environmental signals from your mother and the environment, and then the programming occurs from zero to one."

What was the program that you got in utero? Oh, you don't know that one? Okay, well, how about the program you got from zero to one? You don't know that either, and you say no consciousness was even working. You have no memory of these programs in your conscious mind. From zero to one, from one to two, from two to three, around the age of three you might remember something. You don't remember in utero. You don't remember one being one, two, or three. This means you don't know what your subconscious programs were. And you don't know that because it's not in the conscious mind.

Ninety-five percent of your life is coming from subconscious programs as a fact of science. That's because 95% of your life you're thinking, and while you're thinking, you engage automatic subconscious autopilot programs. And so, this 95% of your life comes from the programs. Your life is a printout of your programs. Here's something you can do to attract the things that you want into your life.

What you have in your life is there because you have programs to acknowledge it. But the things you want, desire, or wish for seem to be a struggle. You put a lot of work into making things happen. Then you say, "I'm pushing, but I'm going to make it happen." Why are you working so hard? Inevitably, the program you've downloaded does not support that outcome. And you're trying to override a 95% program with a 5% conscious program. The subconscious mind is a billion times more powerful than a computer. Mathematically, your conscious mind is not going to take this thing over like that. It doesn't work that way. And this is a problem. We all have educated, conscious minds of "Oh my god, yes! To have good health, let's do physical things. Let's eat well." That's a conscious mind but that's only 5% of your day. Ninety-five percent of your day didn't come from that belief at all.

You could be super smart in the conscious mind and not change one thing in the program of the subconscious mind. A lot of people kid themselves with, "If I become aware of my issues, then I'll know what to change in my life." Many people have read self-help books or gone to lectures and all that stuff, they can learn all about quantum physics, but has their life changed? In most cases, no, it hasn't changed at all. The reason is this, their life is not coming from the conscious mind, it's coming from the subconscious program.

The movie, *The Matrix*, is not science fiction. *The Matrix* is a documentary. Why? All humans have been programmed to function. Like, you might be thinking, "Oh, so I've been programmed?" Here's the cool part about the movie. In the movie, you get a choice of a blue pill or a red pill. When they say the blue pill and you take it, you wake up and you're in the program life. This is just the way it has always been. But if you take the red pill, you get out of the program. And what would that mean?

We're going to tell you because it's recognized that when we fall in love seriously, that is the equivalent of the red pill. You stop thinking because when you fall in love, you stay present, it's not the time to think; you've been looking for this person your whole life. We understand that when people fall in love, they stay mindful, meaning they don't think. If you're not thinking, you're not defaulting to the program. And if you're not thinking, then your conscious mind is in total control. Every day your life is blah, blah, blah, blah, blah, blah, blah. Then you meet somebody

74

and 24 hours later life is not blah blah blah anymore. Life becomes beautiful. You feel so in love, and your life seems like heaven on earth. Everything is wonderful. You feel healthy, happy, and full of joy. When people stop playing the program, they start creating from wishes and desires. Their wishes and desires manifest, and that is the honeymoon. The honeymoon is heaven on earth. It was always there. Except if your subconscious is running the show, then there is no honeymoon program in there.

That's the struggling program. And so, the wake-up call is this from quantum physics. The most valid science acknowledges that consciousness is creating our life experience. Epigenetics, the revolution in biology, reveals that consciousness is creating your genetic and behavioral character. Why is all this relevant? Because we believe we are victims when we are creating every bit of this. And the idea is, if you want to change, take the red pill/change the programs. Changing the programs is not always easy. The reason is that the programs are habits. And if a habit could just change, it's not a habit. Habits do not want to change. Because if they change, by definition, they're not habits. To change the subconscious mind, you can't just think about it. "Oh, I got a new vision, I want everything to be healthy and happy. Today, I'm going to be that happy guy. I'm going to get the best job. All will be wonderful." And I say, "That doesn't change anything." That's just a belief that will operate 5%.

There are very specific ways to change subconscious programming. The first thing we had to do is identify the programs. The easiest way to identify them is to notice what you are struggling with. It's not because the universe won't give it to you, you're struggling because your program is compromising you.

75

Once you figure out what programs are compromising you and determine to change them, how do you do this? Start with not thinking about it but thinking about your conscious mind. And deciding consciously that you want to change a habit. There are only three ways to change the subconscious. Well, there are actually four ways but I going to eliminate one. Why? Because sometimes a circumstance is an accident. In other words, a person might go to a doctor and get a prognosis of terminal cancer. They can change their life right there in that spot because of that news. That could cause them to say, "I've got to change my life." Okay, but there are some things in life that you can't control, and this is an example.

We then have three types of situations that are controllable.

Number one, the first seven years of your life. You were programmed because your mind was in theta, which is hypnosis. There are a whole range of vibrations in the mind. The highest one is beta. We're use this in conversation. When you go home and you relax in the evening, the vibration slows down. It's called alpha; this is calm consciousness. But the moment you fall asleep, the alpha vibrations stop, and now we're in theta vibrations, which is hypnosis. Put earphones on, play a program of something you want to be true in your life. While you're awake, you'll hear some of the programs. But the moment you fall asleep, guess what, the program is coming in, your conscious mind doesn't hear a damn thing because it's sleeping. But the subconscious mind is open, beta. And that's called self-hypnosis- reprogramming yourself at night.

Number two, self-hypnosis gives us programs until age seven, but we still get programs after that. You learn how to drive, it's a program. Oh, how did I learn programs after age seven? The answer was repetition, practice repeated over and over again. If you're not happy but want to be, you can do this. You can just come into your mind right in the middle of not being happy, and just say "I am happy, I am happy." The subconscious mind moves by repetition. If you repeat this continuously, you'll wake up one day, and the subconscious mind will also wake up to, "I'm happy." It's got a program, it's a habit. You're already happy. That's the second reason the new age talk is called, "fake it until you make it." Pretend what you want has happened already, repeat the pretending, and the subconscious will record it as a program.

Lastly, this is the most important one at this moment because human civilization is facing an evolutionary crisis. We have to change behavior. There's a new form of psychology called energy psychology. This involves super learning. Maybe seeing somebody read a book by moving their finger down the page looks like fast reading. As they move their finger down, they read every word on that page. They can sit in the bookstore and five minutes by turning a page, turning a page, turning, they could read the entire book. If you could engage in super learning as a practice, then you can download new behavior virtually instantaneously. Energy psychology modality generally engages super learning.

Why is this relevant? I can change the program in minutes! The first two, the self-hypnosis and the repetition, are both a time-based repetition process. But energy psychology can change a belief in minutes. I have on my website, www.brucelipton.com, about 25 or more modalities of energy psychology with website connections and a little description of each. Look through this list and find one that feels good. Then try it because you can change your belief in 15-20 minutes or less. But you must engage that super learning character for it to download instantly.

You ask, "Can I really change?" Absolutely. What do you want to change? Look at your life and tell yourself where you're struggling. Now, make and repeat a statement that is the positive side of what you're missing. By repeating that statement or energy psychology, you can download that belief in minutes and walk away different. The whole problem with what's going on here is that people believe they're victims. The truth is, each one of us is a creator. But, if you believe you're a victim and believe the Biology of Belief, then because you think you're a victim, then you are. Henry Ford said, "Whether you think you can or whether you think you can't. You're right." This says that your belief is going to manifest in your life. Look at your life. If it's not working the way you want it, don't try to change the world; go inside, and change the beliefs.

We believe that Lifestyle Medicine and health coaching need to be in every clinic, in every health center, in every hospital, and in every doctor's office, because that's how we make a big change. Changing habits are not necessarily easy but having somebody who coaches you would make it so much easier. Your beliefs control this, it's called the placebo effect. The placebo effect says, "I believe this pill, or I believe this therapy is what I need." And you take the pill. You do the therapy. And you get better. Then you find out the pill was a sugar pill. The therapy was a fake, a sham, but it healed you. It wasn't the pill, or the therapy. Placebo is the science of how the mind controls the biological expression of healing. And everybody agrees to the placebo effect that positive thinking can affect your life.

Now, let me tell you the most important part which is left out in these discussions. Negative thinking is equally powerful when controlling your life, but it works in the opposite direction. Negative thinking can cause you to have any disease on this planet and negative thinking can cause you even to die just because you believe you're going to die. If you discard negative thinking, then only positive thinking is going on. Most of your day, you're probably not thinking positive, you're negatively thinking, and your expression is a consequence of your thought because consciousness is creating this. If we leave out negative thinking from a diagnosis or prognosis, then we have missed perhaps the biggest health challenge. It's not in our physiology.

When people are unconscious for a long time and they're in a hospital on machines, their rhythm and metabolism are just beautiful, and everything is working just fine. The moment they wake up, it blows the harmony out of it because all of a sudden, they put the mind back in. The body by itself takes care of itself. It is intelligent beyond anything humans can deal with. That's our problem. Because of our hubris, we think we know more than our biology. It is claimed that humans are brilliant, the top of the pile with everything less than human being less intelligent. You get smaller and smaller animals, less and less intelligent, all the way down to cells. Then it's said that cells are not intelligent. I say, "They created us. Everything in this human body came from a community of cells. Their intelligence supersedes our intelligence." Yet people look down on them and go, "Oh cells are stupid. That's why we need medicine."

Cells aren't stupid. The drivers have had bad driver education. With better driver education we have to re-educate who we are, how we operate, and how powerful we are. Stop telling people that they're victims. Let's empower them.

We must wake up.

We have been sleep-walking through life with our conscious minds drifting out in space somewhere, and our bodies and program moving forward. It's time to bring our "conscious" back into the game because it is the source of empowerment. We must get out of the victim mentality and start to recognize we are the masters of our creation. If everybody wanted to, they could have a forever honeymoon. And if everybody on the planet had a honeymoon right now, it would be heaven on earth.

Chapter Six

Drs. Ayesha and Dean Sherzai – Building Healthy Brains

Team Sherzai are leading doctors and researchers focused on building healthy brains, and authors of "The 30-Day Alzheimer's Solution." Dr. Dean is a behavioral neurologist/ neuroscientist with a Ph.D. in Healthcare Leadership from Loma Linda University. Dr. Ayesha is completing her Ph.D. in Women's Leadership at Columbia University. ↗ teamsherzai.com

This is an incredibly important topic for the world. Brain health is health. We are our brains. We like to joke with the cardiologist and nephrologist that the rest of the body is there to carry the brain. We can replace a kidney and we are still the same person. We can also replace the heart, but we can't replace the brain because that's our personality. That's ourselves, our passions, and our love. That's everything that we are, yet we haven't gotten a good understanding of this amazing brain until the last few decades, when we truly began to realize the power of this brain and the fact that we have control over it. Not in some weird biohacking or superfood, but in a very comprehensive, real way. People in their homes, with their families and their communities, or in their jobs, can do small, incremental changes that can profoundly affect this brain.

Now, this brain is three pounds and 2% of the body's weight. That's small, yet it consumes 25% of your body's energy. That's why the brain needs rest. That's why the brain, more than any other organ, needs the right foods. That's why the brain needs the kind of activity that helps it grow well into your 60s, 70s, 80s, and beyond. There are examples of those kinds of people that have lived into their 80s and 90s and their brains were more functional, more astute, and sharper than even when they were younger.

That's a reality. We develop more and more three-dimensional thinking, but if we don't take care of the brain, then the damage that accumulates appears in our 40s, 50s, and definitely in our 60s and 70s. We have to take care of it.

Here's the secret.

You don't have to pay anybody all kinds of money for vitamin concoctions. They don't have to find a hole in your supplement intake so that they can fill it with their drugs. You don't have to go to some guru. You don't even have to buy our books, although it helps us, and also has some science-based guidance. You do have to bring the changes into your home. The results are remarkable. We have worked on people like Jane Goodall, and Dr. Ellsworth who did open to close surgery and cardiothoracic surgery at age 95. These are incredible examples of cognitive longevity. There are many, many others.

The majority of the population starts their decline, believe it or not, in their 30s.

But we can grow our capacity. Our job is to avoid mild cognitive impairment (MCI) and dementia which overwhelms a significant percentage of the population. In the United States alone, 6.2 million people suffer from Alzheimer's which is a type of Dementia. Dementia is a big category, and Alzheimer's is one type. Alzheimer's is the fastest-growing epidemic beyond COVID. Every 64 seconds, somebody gets diagnosed. It's becoming the number one epidemic in the United States. It is already number one in Japan, and number one in the UK and other countries. We must stop it. The numbers are that one in nine people over 65 suffer from Alzheimer's. African Americans and minority communities are also disproportionally affected. It has a lot to do with socio-economics status, and access to information and good health. The cost is overwhelming. The male to female ratio is quite significant, women suffer twice as much as men.

We have to get rid of some myths.

- Number one is that it cannot be prevented. Nowadays, that is accepted. But when I first spoke about this 15 years ago, it was very controversial. It's no longer controversial and people do understand that you can prevent it. The numbers do vary. Some people say as much as 40% or 50% can be prevented. We say as much as 90%. It's becoming increasingly evident that if you live a true comprehensive healthy lifestyle, it will be 90%.
- The second myth is that the disease starts when you start forgetting. No, the disease process, which is not just Alzheimer's, but cognitive aging starts years and decades earlier. At that point, you don't see the effect because you have some resilience but then all of a sudden in your 60s you start noticing it. The process has started earlier. I want young people to realize that the simple things you do in life can profoundly protect your brain.
- The third myth is that medicine is going to solve this problem. Not with brain diseases. It's not going to be one medicine; it's going to be a more comprehensive approach.
- The fourth myth is that it is a genetic disease. Some diseases have 100% penetrance. Meaning that if you have the genes, you're going to get the disease. Huntington's is one of those, and sickle cell is another. For the great majority of aging diseases, it's a combination of genes, environment, and lifestyle. In Alzheimer's and dementia, it's especially lifestyle. Only 3% of Alzheimer's is driven by genes and if you have the genes, you're going to get the disease no matter what. The rest are lower-level genetic influences, meaning that they have some influence, but it's the environment and lifestyle that have the greater influence.

What are the mechanisms? The mechanisms are inflammation, oxidation, glucose dysregulation, and lipid dysregulation. These are the mechanisms for most brain diseases. This comes from many different directions, but in totality, it's mostly if somebody has uncontrolled diabetes then they are going to have cognitive decline and ultimately dementia. If they have high cholesterol levels for years and years that are uncontrolled, that will affect brain disease. The data is profound. Even mildly elevated cholesterol levels increase your risk of Alzheimer's by 57%. If you have inflammation for long periods, you will have a high risk of dementia.

What do you do to get rid of that? Lifestyle.

The things that affect it are nutrition, exercise, unwinding or stress management, restorative sleep, not just being knocked out with medicines, and optimizing mental activity. We came up with our own, self-serving acronym N.E.U.R.O.; Nutrition, exercise, unwind, restorative sleep, and optimizing mental activity. If people truly incorporate these things extensively into their life, they will avoid the majority of the brain diseases that come with aging.

Even the Alzheimer's Association has been focusing so much on figuring out a medication. In 2019 they came up with the statement that lifestyle factors are the best and the only bet now for reducing dementia risk. This has been proven with large population studies such as this one. This study looked at a pool of populations having the genetic risk for dementia, and they found that they carry a 60% higher risk of developing dementia if they had the genetic risk. However, the same pool of population, when they had an unhealthy lifestyle, their risk went up by 360%.

That's the profound effect of lifestyle on genetic risk and the development of dementia. Then, flipping and looking at a healthy lifestyle, the risk in the same population pool fell to less than

30%. Adherence to a healthy lifestyle can significantly offset genetic risk even if we have the genes. Lifestyle can modify the outcome and we can avoid this devastating disease.

Here is another study that was recent published by the National Institute on Aging. They looked at lifestyle factors, which included nutrition, exercise, cognitive activity, alcohol, smoking, and some other significant factors. We call these NEURO. They found that compared to those who never adhere to any of these healthy lifestyles, such as eating, healthy exercising, etc., those who adhere to two to three lifestyle factors reduce the risk of Alzheimer's disease by 37%.

If they adhere to four to five of these factors, they were able to reduce their risk of Alzheimer's by 60%. That is huge. We're talking about not even perfect adherence, but very moderate adherence to a healthier lifestyle can offset that risk. Prevention is the treatment.

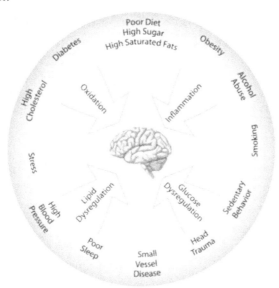

We are not anti-medication, and hopefully, we will have medications for this disease. Currently, we have this incredible opportunity and resource: lifestyle. This preventive mode is helping us lower the risk of this disease and devastating communities.

These four processes are a good pictorial of what leads to Alzheimer's and other dementias. These are the lifestyle variables that affected our nutrition, exercise, unwinding, restorative sleep, and optimizing mental activity. Let's start with nutrition.

Nutrition is probably the most important risk factor because it's the internal environment that we create.

Multiple studies have shown that people who consume an unprocessed plant-based or at least plant predominant diet, tend to do better when compared to a diet with saturated fats which are found in animal products, meat, dairy, cheese, and even coconut oil. A healthier plant-based diet would consist of legumes, whole grains, nuts, seeds, and lots of green leafy vegetables. Healthy fats are obtained from nuts, seeds, and polyunsaturated fats such as extra virgin olive oil. Looking at different dietary factors such as the mind, Mediterranean or the DASH diet can be beneficial diets to keep. The unifying factors between these dietary patterns are the fact that they consist of whole, plant-based foods.

There's so much overlap between these diets and unfortunately, there's a lot of diet wars going on in our communities for unfounded reasons. We all know that incremental movement towards adding more unprocessed plant-based foods results in better brain health and lower risk of not only Alzheimer's disease but also vascular diseases of the brain such as stroke. Fats derived from nut seeds are better because of the poly and monounsaturated fats. Proteins derived from lentil, bean, and soy products like tofu and tempeh are much better. Complex carbohydrates are also a healthy food.

Nobody should be anti-carbohydrates.

There are good carbohydrates, and the brain prefers carbohydrates as a source of fuel. Focusing on increasing our fiber content is incredibly important. Not only do they reduce bad cholesterol, but they provide glucose in a small, viable way, making sure that the brain is not deprived of the multi-variant vitamins and micronutrients that are present in plant-based foods and healthy fats.

As far as exercise goes, nobody fights about exercise because we all agree that it's very important.

It's profoundly important for the brain because when we exercise, regular, moderate to strenuous activity grows the brain. We have studies done on many different populations, showing that people who engage in a regimented exercise program have bigger brains. There's a part of the brain called the hippocampus which is responsible for encoding memory, and that keeps growing as we age and engage in exercise. On the other hand, sedentary behavior completely nullifies the benefits of any exercise program, whether it's moderate or strenuous. Continuously moving is important.

One interesting fact that comes from different studies shows that people who have stronger legs have bigger brains. That could be a funny statement, but if you look at it, bigger legs, bigger brains, it's true and why is that? It's because the biggest muscles in our body are in our legs and when we exercise, we create more growth hormones. There's a specific type of growth hormone called the brain-derived neurotrophic factor which incrementally increases when we engage in exercise. That's essentially a growth hormone for the brain.

The brain cells can make as little as two connections between each other or as many as 30,000 connections. That's the profound capacity of the brain and we can continuously increase that with exercise. People who do both cardio and strengthening exercises have a bigger hippocampus and a lower risk of developing Alzheimer's disease. One study showed that people who had pre-Alzheimer's or the mild cognitive impairment stage were able to reverse MCI. So, it's really important to exercise regularly.

Unwind is essentially stress management.

Stress Management is critically important. We don't make a big deal out of it although we talk about meditation and mindfulness. In reality, we don't talk about it a great deal because people think we don't have control over it. They don't think it has that much of an effect, but it does. In our body, we have two states. One is the survival state (the sympathetic survival state) and then the thriving state which is parasympathetic.

It is not often that we are in a parasympathetic state. Especially in our western lives, we are under constant stress. That stress state was supposed to be used only once in a while, say, when you're running away from a lion. It was beneficial for that one time but then you went back to your parasympathetic state, the restorative and reproducing state.

The reality is, now we live in a constant subclinical level of the sympathetic state where through your limbic hypothalamic-pituitary system, or your limbic hypothalamic endocrine system, you constantly bombard the body with survival state mechanisms, which are not beneficial long term. They are extremely detrimental long term. Cortisol in short bursts is fine, but constant higher levels of cortisol, constant lowering of the immune system, constant lowering of growth hormones, constant lowering of other sex hormones, are going to be incredibly detrimental for the body in general. It will be especially detrimental for the brain, which needs so much help maintaining itself past the age of 30 and 40.

Stress must be managed. The way you manage it is this: divide it into good and bad stress. There is good stress. That's why you have a brain. The brain wants to be challenged, the brain wants to be stressed, and pushed but around its purpose and with clear timelines, goals, and successes. Your dopamine system is there to create addiction towards good stress. As it happens, it also creates bad habits, bad stress, all of that. We can create a pathway of good stress. We have written about this and we're doing an entire other series on good stress and bad stress. If we can identify the good stressors specifically and measurably, and work towards increasing them systematically, then identify the bad stressors specifically and measurably, and reduce, eliminate, delegate, we would have done more benefit for your brain than anything else, because you will have lowered that constant state of sympathetic survival.

The next one is Restore, which is essentially restorative sleep.

Dean and I always say it's the most important time of the day because evolutionarily, we put ourselves in a state of complete unconsciousness. After all, it's that important for the brain. Two very important things happen when we sleep. Firstly, cleansing of the brain through a dedicated janitorial system, which includes the lymphatic system and the microglia (a type of brain cells that pick up the debris and throws it out of the body). Secondly, memory consolidation and organization.

People who are sleep deprived, or have erratic sleep cycles, or have sleep disorders such as sleep apnea and restless leg syndrome, don't reach the deep stages of sleep where memory consolidation and cleansing of the brain habits happens. This significantly increases the risk for Alzheimer's disease.

Another is the Optimization of cognitive activity. Optimizing cognitive activity is profoundly important. There are about 87 billion neurons, each of them making a couple of connections versus 30,000 connections per neuron. Imagine! That power is not like when your body builds and you're the world's greatest bodybuilder, maybe you doubled your size. In this case, you're multiplying 15,000 times. Of course, it's not exactly that.

Optimizing is about good stress. Find one or multiple purposes, push yourself and challenge yourself around those purposes, that's how you make those connections. That's the highest level of plasticity and growth for the brain. We know that people who are higher educated are significantly protected against Alzheimer's. Not always, but in general and by numbers. It's not education that causes this, it has to do with people who have pushed themselves with their businesses, with their music, with their dancing, and with their organizations.

Optimizing is about finding your purpose, pushing yourself, challenging yourself, and building that brain to the point that it gives you resilience against everything.

A few books we wrote, "*The Alzheimer Solution*" in 2017, and our latest book that came out in March of 2021, is "*The 30-day Alzheimer's solution.*" We talked about the neuro plan and the latest evidence-based medicine on the prevention of Alzheimer's disease. We would love to keep in touch with everyone on social media, and we invite you to take a look at our Healthy Minds initiative, which is our non-profit. It essentially provides all these resources for different communities to take care of their brain health.

The realization that brain health is so important is starting to expand. The question of needing a ketogenic diet for Alzheimer's, brain health, and the brain-eating ketones to function comes in. A lot of people have that kind of concept. However, we go by evidence. We don't just go by anecdotal evidence, short, small data evidence, or six months of evidence. There are no long-term data for this and no population-based long-term data. We are completely open to research whatever direction it takes. The field of ketogenic research comes from neurology for patients that had uncontrolled seizures.

With medication, they put them on a ketogenic diet, which made ketones. It's a type of seizure only found in children, Lennexia Gastroenterol. They helped reduce the frequency, but that's during a shocking state. It's like saying because chemotherapy helps cancer patients, we should all take chemotherapy, NO. That line of argument should stop. Where it is shown beneficial outside of that is nominal, weak, and non-reproducible, and never produced long term. As public health people, we say if it can't be generalized to the population, it cannot be applied.

People don't understand that the majority of people who do a ketogenic diet never really get into ketosis because it's difficult to maintain ketosis. It's extremely difficult. The data is very weak. We have never seen strong enough data. Not large enough study, or long enough study to show benefit.

Most of the outcomes for the short studies in very few people who had advanced Alzheimer's disease do not even show improvement in global cognitive scores. They showed the people felt good, but it didn't change their cognitive scores. You always feel good if you have a lot of attention on you. I could probably smile at someone and make them feel good. There are a lot of flaws in the way that research has been described.

On the other hand, we have a tremendous amount of evidence showing that people who eat more vegetables, fruits, and unprocessed plant-based foods reduce the risk of disease. Ignoring all of that and trying to hone in on a very weak source of data is interesting.

We have data coming to us from the mind diet, Mediterranean diet and stroke, and the Adventist Health Study. When you look at all of them or do factor analysis, the component that comes back over and over strongly is a plant-centered diet. Even if you're not going to go plant pure, a mostly plant-based diet that cleanses from processed food is incredibly protective.

You have a humongous weight of truth on this side, decades and decades of Framingham Study, the Rush Study, and the Adverse Health Study. Let us say 50 years of large data shows that a plant-centered diet protects you from dementia as much as 50 to 60%. Yet, on this side, you have almost no data. Why? Well, it is because people love hearing good news about their bad habits. It's a meat-driven argument. Everybody is so passionate about this. It's very dogmatic. I think that is part of what we tried to do just for us to step above it and say that is 80% of what we probably all agree upon, and not just the one to 3% that we want to fight about.

There is the question about Restorative Sleep.

A lot of people don't know the importance of restorative sleep, especially the cleansing of the brain aspect. We activate a very interesting system when we enter the third stage of sleep. We have the first stage, second stage, third stage, and then REM sleep. In the third stage, there are these cells called microglia that get activated and they go around the brain, and they start picking up debris.

There's also a lymphatic system which is lymph — a fluid that essentially flushes the brain and gets rid of these accumulated byproducts which include amyloid protein. Amyloid protein has been associated with Alzheimer's disease. People who have disrupted sleep architecture, not only do not activate the system, but these microglia go awry. They start eating away at the healthy part of the brain. People who have sleep disorders have shrunken brains. They have brain atrophy because these microglia start eating away at the most important structural elements of the brain.

Sleep hygiene is very important. It helps us ensure that we rule out problems like sleep apnea and restless leg syndrome or any other disruption or mechanism that disrupts sleep. They've also done studies to show that people who don't have enough sleep have poor memory regardless of any pathology. These processes can even disrupt our attention, focus, learning information, processing information, and making good decisions.

We have experienced that ourselves. When we don't sleep, we don't make good judgments. We make really bad decisions. We have to make sure we learn more and more about it. That's why it's important to include this into comprehensive, multifaceted lifestyle for brain and general health.

I want the doctors and the healthcare workers to realize that the concept that stops us from actually getting into this is the a priori belief that people can't change themselves and medicine can change them. That comes from the fact that we didn't have good methods of behavior change. We just throw things at people to be motivated. Pick yourself up by the bootstraps.

Now, through behavioral science and behavioral neurology, we know that small, incremental, measurable, and goal-directed behaviors become cumulative. It becomes additive, multiplicative, and a complete health and behavior change model that empowers the person even beyond their lifestyle components.

By focusing on small, measurable, incremental changes that you agree with the person around their capacities and weakness, and strengths, you empower them. Not just with that thing, but in their entire life behavioral model changes. That's incredible power and it takes three minutes.

John, how are you doing? What would you like to change about yourself?

"Oh, I have a little extra weight."

Okay, great. In your food systems, which one do you think is bad? Is it the foods that are affecting your sugar or processed meat or maybe white bread?

"I eat a lot of white bread."

Okay, great. Then let's just focus on white bread. Next week, find out how much white bread you are eating. That's it, that's your job. Okay.

Then coming back, what you do is for the next month. You eliminate white bread and replace it with wheat bread or reduce it by half that rate of consumption. This is measurable, attainable, and time-bound for the next month. Your dopamine system is designed for that behavior. Your dopamine system is a reward system built around expectations. By the few expectations they achieve, they create an entire wave of behavior change. If they fail because you told them to just be healthy, then you've created an entire negative dopamine and serotonin system.

Here is a magical concept. Focus on either white bread or sugar but pick one of them. By specifically and measurably changing your life around that, you've changed your entire neurotransmitter relationship with joy, happiness, success, habits, addiction, etc.

We call that prescribing lifestyle medicine.

Chapter Seven

Dr. David Perlmutter – Alzheimer's, Dementia, and Brain Health

Dr. Perlmutter is a Board-Certified Neurologist and five-time New York Times bestselling author of <u>Grain Brain</u> and <u>Drop Acid</u>. He serves on the Board of Directors and is a Fellow of the American College of Nutrition. ↗ drperlmutter.com

My mission as a neurologist has certainly evolved over time. Early in my neurology career, I was focused on basically treating symptoms. I became dissatisfied because I felt that I was treating the smoke but ignoring the fire. I took it upon myself to do the best I could to explore what the heck was causing the brain to go bad. I set out to focus on offering people a fighting chance in a world where there is no treatment for brain failure, Alzheimer's, or other forms of dementia. To this day, we do not have any meaningful treatment whatsoever. It's vital for us to look at what is going on. Are there ways to prevent some of these brain issues?

I made this my mission about 25 years ago. When I set out, I learned there was a lot of information available, even back then.

Over the years our need for this information has compounded. Many have realized the impact that lifestyle choices make in relation to our brain health. Brain health is optimal functionality with a strong resistant to disease.

We talk about lifestyle choices, and how they relate to heart disease and other health risks like diabetes, and cancer. But we rarely talk about brain health.

Over the past three decades I've learned that lifestyle choices have a huge impact on the brain, such as:

- Foods that we eat
- Food that we avoid
- The amount of sleep we get
- The quality of sleep that we get
- Exercise
- Stress

Each of these areas are vitally important in influencing the brain and its operation from moment to moment. One important question I asked was, "What is the brain's risk for degeneration long-term?"

I was able to find a large body of science to support the fact that our everyday choices really have an impact on charting our brain's destiny. This is very empowering.

Our daily habits are important to improving our brain health. Without ranking them, I'm going to start with the importance of sleep. Sleep has an incredibly powerful impact on keeping our brains healthy. Lack of sleep is known to be damaging to the brain and our overall health. The quality of sleep, as well as the length of sleep, is just as important.

A strong risk factor for brain decline is lack of quality sleep. Without the brain going into deep sleep, or REM (Rapid eye movement), lack of sleep puts the body at higher risk for not only brain degeneration, but also diabetes, cancer, heart disease, weight gain, and depression, to name a few.

For example, if you are type 2 diabetic, you may have as much as a quadrupled risk for Alzheimer's. Can you see how the body is all related? Both of these health issues share common mechanisms, for example, inflammation. It seems important to "shine the light on" sleep issues and how this relates to our overall health. Sleep is one of the most underrated lifestyle habits that we need to look at. Questions we might want to start with are, "How do we measure our sleep?" and, "How can we go about getting a better night's sleep?" We will come back to this after exploring more about the importance of sleep and sleep quality.

Food, exercise, even water, we can go without for a while. But sleep, we can't, without collapsing.

And after a few nights without sleeping, you cannot even survive. This has been proven with laboratory animals. It is difficult to say how much each person needs for a quality night's rest, but most indicators point to around eight hours. Remember, I also mentioned the quality of sleep is just as important as the quantity. This brings us to more questions in understanding the value of our sleep.

- Do you fall asleep quickly?
- Do you wake up many times during the night?
- Do you have restless legs at night while trying to sleep?
- Do you need to go to the bathroom during the night?
- Does your partner snore at night and keep you awake?
- Are there disturbing outdoor noises while you are trying to sleep?
- Do you ever feel like you don't reach the deep or REM phase of sleep?
- How do you really know when you are sleeping or when you're awake?

It's important to understand REM and deep sleep, and how much you get each night. During deep sleep, the brain cleans itself. This is called the glymphatic systems wherein the brain purges itself of accumulated toxins of the day. For example, these accumulated toxins could be proteins misfolding, viruses, or other toxins that the brain wants to rid itself of. Without going into deep sleep, this reduction or elimination of toxins won't happen. This is very detrimental to your brain short-term as well as long-term.

The good news is, we now have user-friendly technology available to track our sleep quality and quantity. I personally use a device called Oura Ring. There are many of these types of devices. They are all fairly standard with the type of information they can provide regarding your sleep and sleep patterns. Some of the most important results you want to be able to track are:

- How much sleep did you get?
- How long did it take you to fall asleep?
- How much time did you spend in deep sleep and REM sleep?

With the results of a sleep tracker we can make better decisions for lifestyle choices and changes. Let me give you a personal example of this. About three weeks ago, I had another vaccine for COVID, and I didn't tolerate it very well. When I first got home, I thought everything was great. But towards the evening, I developed a high fever of 104° F. This is especially high for me. My sleep that night, as you might expect, was very bad. That morning my sleep tracker showed a total sleep score in the upper 60s, which is unheard of for me; I generally have very good sleep. The "sleep score" is based on a rating of 1-100.

The next night I still had a temperature of 104° F and another bad night's sleep. The next day my fever broke and I began feeling better. I regained my energy, started to run again, exercise, do all the things I normally do, and I felt fine. But my sleep scores were still bad and stayed bad for several nights. During this time I was taking some melatonin, going to sleep earlier, eating a little bit earlier, and just playing with different variables to see what I could do to get my sleep back on track.

After making many different changes, I found that shifting my exercise from the morning to the late afternoon or early evening, made a huge difference. I woke up the next day with a score of 96 and feeling like a new person.

This might not be specifically what everybody needs to do, but with a sleep tracker, each individual can figure out their best personal habits. It may be eating less in the evening, eating earlier, limiting blue light exposure, sometimes making a room quieter or darker can help, or even sleeping in a different room. There are many variables we can look at clearly with the aid of a sleep-tracker. Many of these trackers even allow us to get printed reports when the software syncs up with our computer.

Another area of restorative sleep that we should look at is its association with an increase level of beta-amyloid in the brain. This type of protein is associated with Alzheimer's disease. Although some research challenges this, most confirms a relationship. One of the symptoms of this buildup of protein in the brain is increased impulsiveness. We all know how this creates poor choices, especially when related to food, and thus compounding an already unhealthy situation. Even one night of bad sleep can cause a person to make poor food decisions the following day. You're tired, you eat whatever is convenient, and usually highly refined carbohydrate comfort foods. This ultimately leads to weight gain, which can lead to sleep problems including sleep apnea.

Can you see the vicious cycle this could lead to? And we know that obesity is associated with Alzheimer's, diabetes, cancer, heart disease, and other serious health issues.

Paying attention to your sleep is a good way to help you pay attention to your health. You can discover what choices influence your sleep patterns and how you feel during the day. Setting up a good strategy helps you become aware of what variables you can changes or adjust to improve sleep and nutrition.

We are fortunate to live in a time where we have tools that give us precise and immediate feedback in terms of the effects of changes on our physiology.

I've suggested wearing sleeping devices to give us a look at sleeping patterns each morning. These devices can connect with our smart phones and computer, and provide information on our heart rate, heart rate variability, and sleep patterns. The software then keeps a running log for months so you can refer back to your long-term sleeping patterns. This is all good information.

Another helpful health device is the Continuous Glucose Monitor (CGM). This is a small patch that you wear on your left shoulder. This collects blood sugar information to your smartphone and gives regular readings throughout the day. Tracking your blood sugar levels throughout the day is fundamental to your health. With the collected information, you can make changes and see how they impact your health. For example, some particular foods are not healthy for you, but you might not be aware of it.

Doctor visits with fasting blood sugar readings are also a way to measure and track CGM, but this gives hindsight versus up-to-the-moment results. Having a dynamic, real-time understanding of your blood sugar related to your lifestyle can be extremely helpful. Questions you can ask yourself for gaining a better understanding of your sleep patterns could be:

- What impact does a bad night's sleep have on my blood sugar the following day?
- Did I sleep as well last night as I feel I did?
- How is my blood sugar level looking over time?
- What changes can I make to improve my overall health?

100

- How are certain foods impacting my blood sugar levels?
- What foods seem to best help control my blood sugar balance?

Without technology, it is quite difficult to know how to control your blood sugar level. This is a great way to track the impact that food has on our daily blood sugar levels and what foods we can incorporate into our lives to make positive changes. To sum it up, making improvements to our daily blood sugar level is about making changes in the foods we eat.

Let's look next at the timing of our day-to-day activities as this is also very important in optimizing our health. I've mentioned the timing of activities as it relates to sleep. For example, shifting exercise to later in the day seemed to work wonders for my sleeping pattern.

The timing of our eating is equally as important. Many studies are now showing that eating within a short window of time each day and causing a longer "fasting" period between food intake, can be healthy. Our metabolic health is influenced by the number of hours in a 24-hour period that we are eating, or conversely, that we are fasting/not eating.

Here are two examples:

- Eating three meals a day - breakfast (7 am), lunch (12 pm), dinner (7 pm).
  - Eating twelve hours on, twelve hours off.
- Time-restricted eating.
  - Eating within an eight-hour span, sixteen hours off, with water all day.

Our typical three meals a day might seem most comfortable but is not as effective to our metabolic health. Time-restricted eating has the better metabolic effects, specifically with blood sugar balance. Controlling blood sugar helps with the regulation of the hormone insulin. This is an exciting technique in helping insulin do its job.

It's quite likely that our genetics connect us back to our hunter-gatherer days when we didn't stop moving during the day. People likely ate once or twice a day, then spent the rest of their awake time moving. Modern science in both laboratory animals and humans confirms this is a good routine. We've been talking about when to eat. Now we'll talk about what to eat.

We have all heard that "breakfast is the most important meal of the day." Let's deconstruct this. Breakfast means "breaking the fast." When is the best time to do this? And does it matter what you have for that meal? In most developed countries, especially in America, people seem to eat the worst foods for breakfast They start off their day with the biggest carb-load you can imagine. Then the rest of the day is downhill from there. What you have for breakfast is one equation of your morning. When you have it is the other. What is the optimum time to "break the fast?" The longer you can put it off in the morning, the better. Ten a.m. would be good, but noon would be even better for your metabolic health.

The timing of your breakfast is also important for detox.

Intermittent fasting or time-restricted eating has many positive impacts on human physiology. Most importantly, it increases what's called "autophagy", or the ability to break down cells and recycle their defective components. We know from animal studies that even short fasts can do this. We don't yet have a good marker on exactly how this impacts humans, but I think it does happen.

There are other pillars of health that are positively impacted by time-restricted eating which include metabolic issues. This would include improved insulin, a decrease in inflammation, and even activation of the body's innate antioxidant and detoxification systems.

Regarding nutrition, most people are fixated, and with good reason, on what they eat. What is incredible to me is how the narrative on this has changed over the past couple of decades. For example, just a few decades ago, fat was the villain, and everyone did whatever they could to eliminate it from their diets. Around the world, we were offered low-fat and no-fat everything, from cookies to yogurt to meats. The message we got was that "fat is evil."

We now understand why that happened. It was a ploy of the sugar industry and its profound impact on us to eat more carbs, higher carbs, and more refined carbs, and this was supposed to be a good thing. The influence that the sugar industry had on peer-reviewed and respected medical journals is a sad story.

These days there is much better review and research. Science is dominant and now says that fasting is an essential part the human diet and has been for thousands of years. During the 1960s and 70s, after an article by Ancel Keys in Time magazine, we were sold a bill of goods that a low-fat diet was healthy. Since that time a lot of research is showing how vital good fats are to our health. Plenty of scary and unhealthy fats have been identified as well as refined carbohydrates; all showing no place in human nutrition.

Did you know that the United States government recommends up to 10% of calories from refined carbohydrates? This is breathtaking since it is in strong contrast with what our best science tells us about keeping our body's insulin balanced. This balance enables the wonderful hormone insulin to be appreciated by the cells in the body so they can answer the door when insulin comes knocking. And then helping to balance our blood sugar level. In addition to this, insulin also sustains the growth and health of our brain cells. The brain contains connections called synapse with a dependency on a good insulin balance and quality fat to develop and function properly.

All of this should lead us to understanding the need for good fats back on the table and into our diets. Fats were always necessary in human diets for health and longevity. Refined carbohydrates, on the other hand, were not. Simple carbs, like sugar, contains whole fructose, helpful in the past as an internal signal to our ancestors. Fructose signals the body to get ready for food scarcity. Late summer and early fall are when food ripens. This is also the time of year that bears get ready for hibernation. Food containing sugar fructose is available then to help them ramp-up for winter. We should take this as an example.

Bears and humans should be aware of their innate warning mechanism that winter is coming. It's time to make more fat in preparation, as well as becoming a little more insulin resistant, so the body and brain can get powered with glucose. This process needs set in motion before we run low of calories and could be at risk of dying from starvation. During the winter months, calories and food are not abundant. The means for survival has worked its way into our genome, even before hunter-gatherer primates. This genetic experience made primates a little fatter and turned on their glucose production for a season. We are the ancestors of the primates, and still have the same mechanism that they did 14-17 million years ago. It was the survival of the fattest, not the fittest. Their storage of fat at the time got them through a couple million years of food scarcity.

We now know that fructose consumption, despite what the high fructose corn syrup lobbyists would have us believe, is staggering. Statistics show the average American ate only two pounds of sugar a year two hundred years ago, the 2021 average is now around 152 pounds per year.

We now understand what we suspected for years, that consuming fructose, drinking soft drinks, eating highly processed sweet deserts, and eating sugar-containing foods all day long, is related to obesity. The obesity then brings about diabetes, increased inflammation in the body, many other health diseases, and issues that we'd all like to avoid.

In the past couple of decades, we've learned that fructose metabolizes in the body into uric acid. Most are familiar with uric acid and its relationship to gout and kidney stones. It's turning out that uric acid, the metabolite of fructose, is also a danger signal to the body. We need to understand the importance to cutting out fructose from our diets in order to control uric acid and its dangers. This includes cutting out alcohol and other sources that compound the uric acid health issues. The breaking down of these products of the DNA and RNA into uric acid is incredible. And it's interesting to now know the ultimate signaling mechanism of how fructose causes the dirty work through the production of uric acid.

This new information is a powerful tool worth more study. The discovery is becoming a central player around the world. Uric acid is no longer thought to be an innocent bystander but a key component to diabetes, metabolic syndrome, hypertension, weight gain, elevated triglycerides, dyslipidemia, blood issues, and various good and bad cholesterol. This is a huge, new, powerful tool in our toolbox. Since we now understand controlling and lowering uric acid through dietary changes, we can positively impact the health of a huge populous.

If a home monitor for uric acid were developed, like the other smart health monitors, we would be able to monitor important parameters and improve metabolic health.

Back to diet, let's look at the variety of them available from vegan to paleo, and Mediterranean to keto. There are so many out there, all with the pros and cons, and with paleo being a little ill-defined. What is the basic premise we want to look at here? We want to honor our Paleolithic genome. And we want to provide genome signals in the form of food to allow healthy genes to express themselves and suppress the genes that would be harmful. Harmful genes create inflammatory chemicals and compromise our antioxidant system while good genes regulate our detoxification system. We want to do all of this while also avoiding an evolutionary environmental mismatch.

Vegan and vegetarianism are based on non-animal food diets. The Mediterranean diet is another well-studied, plant-based diet. Most studies of these types of diets validate risk reduction for dementia, breast cancer, heart disease, and other chronic health diseases.

Some of these diets center around what I call "broad strokes" or looking at just portions of the diet. For example, looking at only carbohydrates. When diets want no or low carbs, they throw out fiber-rich foods, like vegetables and fruits, which have their many health benefits. This isn't what we want to do. We desperately need fiber for a multitude of reasons.

The most important issue with any diet, I would say, is to look at nurturing the gut biome.

This is the core of what our health fully depends on. Having said this, I want to state the importance of grain and grain-derived products, especially whole grains. These foods are a powerful source of carbohydrates that the body breaks down into energy-producing sugars. And remember, the worst foods, from a health perspective, are the refined carbohydrates from sugars and highly processed grains. Be it glucose or fructose, or a combination of the two, they are not a good intake of sugars.

Some will say that fructose is a better sugar than starches or glucose, but why? They would say it's because fructose doesn't need insulin for its metabolism. Therefore, when it comes to consuming fructose, we're not as at risk for diabetes or insulin resistance issues. This logic is bogus. The truth is fructose dramatically increases blood sugar through two mechanisms. First, fructose stimulates glucose in the live. Second, fructose increases uric acid which leads to insulin resistance, and increases blood sugar level. Fructose is anything but a safe sugar. And would this mean we shouldn't eat fruit? No, not at all. "An apple a day keeps the doctor away." But to gorge on fruit all day would be setting you up to hibernate like a bear, stimulating pathways, and increasing the production of body fat.

We don't want to be packing fat on the body but putting it back on the tables. We also want to dramatically be limiting processed carbs, refined carbs, and sugars. But this doesn't mean we want to eliminate carbs that are found with good fiber. These are critically important.

Next to focus on is protein. Protein requirements depends on each individual's level of activity, weight, and other issues. It's a personal needs issue. We could say that an average or reasonable amount would be around 20% of total intake of calories. Some rules regarding protein would apply to everyone, but in general, it is individualized. We call this "personalized medicine" which looks at individual specifics and genetics to determine the best for each person based on their genetic nuances. As important as genetics is each person's microbiome, their activity level, and even seasonal living conditions.

In general, we can say that the biggest dietary problems for most humans are refined carbs and sugars. What humans seem to do well with is a diet with good fats. Tailored exercise is also something that benefits everyone. And then a reminder of the wearable devices that help track activity, glucose, and other daily habits. All these areas can and should be adjusted for each individual.

Some of the key elements of the Lifestyle Medicine Summit are - empowering health professionals, doctors, and physicians to prescribe lifestyle medicine; health coaching; and integrating these ideas into their practices. The Vinay Jing Yellow Emperor in fourth century BC stated that prevention is the ultimate principle of wisdom. To cure a disease after it has manifested is like digging a well after one feels thirsty, or forging weapons when the war has already begun. This is a huge lesson for us all because modern medicine continues fighting wars against one thing or another. In many regards, we are losing battle after battle. We certainly seem to be losing the war as it relates to Alzheimer's disease. The majority of people seemingly focus on one notion solely, like trying to figure out if it's beta-amyloid or whatever it is. And then what kind of drug can be developed. Many are finally starting to figure out this doesn't work as a long-term solution.

That said, we have known for a couple of decades that lifestyle choices have a huge impact on all health issues. Positive lifestyle habits lower risk of all illness and disease. These habits include:

- Regular exercise
- Engagement in active activities that people enjoy
- Practicing stress management
- Monitoring and keeping blood sugar levels moderate
- Weight management

If we can focus on prevention, and keeping people healthy, rather than taking a reactive approach and treating symptoms, we can have much better outcomes. We have evidence to show this is possible. We also know there seems nothing heroic about keeping people healthy from a "medical" standpoint. We see most people want to live their lives haphazardly, then turn to healthcare practitioners to fix them after they become diabetic, clinically obese, or cognitively impaired. We know these issues are all harder to turn around than to just prevent.

The biggest causes of death today are the chronic inflammatory, degenerative diseases- heart disease, diabetes, Alzheimer's, and cancer. What is the common denominator of these that we have control of? It's inflammation. And with teaching people to understand and change this, we can teach empowerment.

We can conclude that it is vitally important for people who are influencers, those respected and involved in healthcare, to get the word out. We can encourage people to pave the way towards healthy, disease-free lives. The way of Lifestyle Medicine is very valuable to short- and long-term health, as well as cost-effective in taking care for yourself and others. And it is also a much kinder way to care for people before they get sick and need fixed.

Chapter Eight

Joel Fuhrman MD – Autoimmune, Inflammatory Bowel, Diabetes, Heart Disease, and More

Joel Fuhrman, M.D., is a board-certified family physician, seven-time New York Times bestselling author, and nutritional researcher who specializes in preventing and reversing disease through nutritional and natural methods. His five PBS shows, Food as Medicine, have raised over $70 million for PBS. ↗ drfuhrman.com

In my childhood and early 20s, I competed in pairs figure skating, and I was third in the World Professional Pair Skating Championships with my sister Gale, in 1976. Unfortunately, I had an injury that put me on crutches for almost a year, so I was not in the 1976 Olympics. Following that, I began working in my family's shoe business. While I was competing in my teenage years, I was always studying nutrition, not only for better stamina and conditioning, but also to prevent getting sick. My father was overweight and sickly, and I was studying a lot of nutrition books with him so he could change his health trajectory. During the 1960s and 70s, nutrition was already a passion and a hobby of mine.

I didn't originally pursue a pre-medical route in college. I was taking courses like economics and business. About five years into it I realized my passion for nutritional healing would be best expressed by going to medical school. From the beginning I wanted to be a physician, specializing in nutritional medicine. First, I attend the postgraduate pre-med program at Columbia to complete my pre-medical requirements. I was then accepted to the University of Pennsylvania School of Medicine, which I attended from 1984 to 1988. Even in my family practice residency, I was treating people in the clinics with nutritional advice. When I finished my residency, I opened my practice. Back then, nutrition was viewed with skepticism by most doctors. I found it tremendously exciting and rewarding to enable people to get well using nutritional practices as a therapeutic modality.

The science has always supported that if we design a dietary portfolio to maximally slow aging, extend human lifespan, and protect against disease, it will also be therapeutically effective in reversing disease.

I have helped many patients with lupus, fibromyalgia, asthma, rheumatoid arthritis, heart disease, diabetes, headaches, and so much more. Surprisingly, most physicians don't sufficiently understand the biology to enable a recovery from a disease like asthma or lupus. They may see that diabetes and heart disease are reversible, but they're not quite versed in the fact that autoimmune diseases can also be reversed, even psoriasis and multiple sclerosis.

Early in my career, I had a 16-year-old female patient with lupus who had a creatinine level of 4.2. She was on the national renal transplant list, waiting for a new kidney, yet she made a complete recovery. Her creatinine went down to 0.8, and she no longer needed a kidney transplant. Her lupus disappeared and she got well. That's just one example of a complete healing that I've seen with my treatment.

I say this with more than 30 years of experience aiding people's recoveries from serious illnesses using nutritional therapy. And not only diabetes and heart disease, but issues such as multiple sclerosis, lupus, rheumatoid arthritis, and connective tissue disease. Deprescribing or weaning patients off medication is so much more satisfying than adding more and more drugs as people get sicker. I love to share this with other doctors. I think one of the things I'm most proud of is helping Lifestyle Medicine doctors who came to work with me early in their careers and shadowed me in my practice, and others who I have influenced to pursue nutritional medicine.

The fact that nutritional courses are not taught in medical school has always been a major issue. This is a strange paradox because although there are many published studies on food, there are many barriers to completing and publishing study data that demonstrate the effectiveness of nutritional protocols to reverse disease. I have described individual case studies in medical journals of people I've helped recover from cancer and autoimmune diseases. It is unfortunately much more challenging to conduct clinical studies because it costs over a million dollars each to do controlled interventional programs. And it very difficult finding funding.

My goal with the Nutritional Research Foundation is to raise money to fund these important disease-reversal studies. I have made progress, but certainly, I have not obtained the funding required for clinical trials that will impact medicine with the necessary degree of significance, such as taking 50 patients with lupus who are following the same protocol and measuring the outcomes. It is too expensive, and I have not yet had the resources to conduct these trials. We don't have the resources of the pharmaceutical industry, nor the support of the government for such investments.

At the University of Pennsylvania, where I went to school, some of the doctors at the Scheie Eye Institute saw many of my patients with diabetic retinopathy and macular degeneration reverse their condition, and no longer require surgeries or laser treatments. The department approached me to do a study with them, so I sat down at a table with ten ophthalmologists who had done a lot of research and received many National Institutes of Health (NIH) grants in the past. We wrote a terrific grant proposal, sent it to the NIH requesting a $1.5 million budget, and the NIH turned it down. When I tried to inquire with more depth into the rejection, I learned that the NIH presumed that the physicians submitting the study proposal hadn't done nutritional research projects in the past, only other eye studies. They only wanted to fund the same researchers they had been funding in the past. They rejected funding this group of physicians doing such a novel nutritional study, regardless of its importance. I still have that rejected proposal. It was an excellent 40-page paper diagramming all the reasons for the study and their recommendations on its value. It was a terrific grant proposal to the NIH that wasn't accepted.

I then approached the diabetes department at the University and their response was, "We know it works and we know that what you do is very effective, but we can't get people to apply it. And we're not going to waste our time trying to convince people to eat a healthful diet; it's just a waste of our time." The medical profession doesn't have the skills, the knowledge, or the training to teach, encourage, and motivate people to change their diets. In order for people to make changes and resolve food addiction, physicians need training, as well as staff development and implementation to support their patients. The reason for failure is that doctors don't know what they don't know, and they haven't even tried. They don't deny that nutritional medicine works, but they believe they couldn't possibly convince people to make the dietary changes necessary. They are right to a degree, because inducing significant dietary intervention is a developed skill, and food addiction is difficult to resolve.

From my experience, I know that people change when they have the right guidance and support. I couldn't be more excited and passionate about my work, even at the age of 68. After all these years in practice, I'm still just as enthusiastic whenever I see a new patient. Today, people come to my retreat for two, three, or four month, to recover from various conditions like fatty liver, autoimmune hepatitis, diabetes, and even psoriasis and psoriatic arthritis, which all predictably go away. It is always inspiring. I see the frustration and even the disappointment of regular medical doctors seeing their patients become sicker and sicker. So often they lose their excitement about their careers because they aren't making a positive impact on their patient's health trajectory, nor do they see their patients recover. They are just managing diseases. Often, they burn out and are unhappy in their careers. This is a subject dear to my heart, and one that I'm very passionate about. So, I am always enthusiastic about young doctors starting careers in Lifestyle Medicine, hoping that they will develop an economically viable practice, and learn the skills to help people in this way.

I was one of the founding members of the American College of Lifestyle Medicine. Early in my career we had a convention with 20 to 30 people in attendance. Now, thousands of doctors and other healthcare practitioners come to these events. Despite the growth in Lifestyle Medicine, most of the public has been brainwashed with the religion of modern medicine that drugs are the answer. The epidemic of disease is a factor of misdirected worship of drugs and pharmaceuticals, combined with the addictive nature of unhealthy foods, and an inherent mindset that thinks change is too difficult. Most of the public continues eating whatever they want to eat. They are not looking for good, nutritional healthcare. Most people are satisfied with conventional medical care where they take drugs for the rest of their lives.

Another problem, with the advent of the internet, is that there is an overwhelming amount of information out there. Everybody has a diet or a nutritional theory to promote. I coined the term "Nutritarian diet" because, foundationally, it describes a diet designed to be optimal for health and lifespan. With certain diseases, we might have to make certain modifications or adjustments, but the foundational principle of the Nutritarian diet is a plant-based diet that's designed to be rich in micronutrients, phytochemicals, and antioxidants. It is also nutritionally complete, and contains the most powerful anti-cancer, longevity-promoting foods. It is a diet heavy in vegetables and not a grain-based diet. It's not a fruit-based diet. It's not a potato-based diet. It's not a macrobiotic or rice-based diet. It's a vegetable-based, nutritionally adequate diet that includes a variety of foods. Reason being, we know now that the more variety of different foods and fibers you consume in your diet, the greater diversity of disease-fighting phytonutrients you receive. This diet also contributes to a more robust microbiome to fight inflammation in the gut.

Many popular plant-based diets are deficient in some respects that make them not optimal. They might be too high-glycemic, or too low in fats. In the vegan movement or the plant-based movement in the United States, a few popular nutritional gurus have advocated taking all fats out of the diet, including nuts and seeds. In its place, people tend to eat more carbohydrates like potatoes, rice, bread, and pasta. But there's an overwhelming amount of uncontroversial and irrefutable evidence, with scores of corroborative studies, showing that eliminating nuts and seeds from a diet increases cardiovascular deaths, cancer deaths, and overall mortality. I recommend the judicious consumption of nuts and seeds, particularly of high omega-3 containing nuts and seeds - flax seeds, hemp seeds, chia seeds, walnuts - especially for those with heart disease or any health condition.

Half of one's daily nut and seed consumption should be from the high omega-3 category, with the remainder from almonds, sunflower and pumpkin seeds, pine nuts, and others. For most, half an ounce of nuts with each meal or about an ounce and a half of nuts per day, is appropriate; however, even greater amounts are beneficial for slim, highly active individuals. In the Adventist Health Study 2, the study population was divided into quintiles by nut and seed consumption. The highest quintile, consuming more than 1.5 ounces per day, had the most protection from heart attacks, and the most longevity. The lowest quintile consumed less than 0.4 ounces per day and had the highest cardiovascular deaths. For most of my overweight patients, approximately half an ounce of nuts and seeds with each meal is a reasonable figure to provide maximum benefits without consuming too many calories. Eating nuts with each meal facilitates the maximal absorption of the fat-soluble vitamins and phytochemicals in vegetables. So, when you're eating nuts and seeds with your salad for lunch, for example, you are absorbing 20 to 50 times as much anti-cancer and immune-supporting phytochemicals than having that salad without them.

For the overweight, based on age, gender, body size, and exercise level, calories are typically kept in the 1200 to 1600 range to ensure weight loss. Older, overweight women tend to lose weight more slowly. Of course, those who do not need to lose weight may need more calories than average, and can increase their nut and seed intake and other foods to meet their caloric needs. Most following my dietary guidance at my retreat drop between 15 and 20 pounds the first few months. One of my retreat patients recently lost 100 pounds in three months during his stay - roughly a pound a day - and he was a guy eating lots of food, but he was also highly active. Our goal is to teach our guests how to make food taste delicious so this becomes the way they prefer to eat, and they can continue to benefit after they leave.

Recently one of our guests weighing 380 pounds, lost 80 pounds during her three-month stay. She then lost 80 more pounds after returning home because of what she learned from us. Ultimately, the goal is not to see how fast people can lose weight. What we're trying to do is provide individuals with the knowledge and emotional skills that they need once they go home. This ideally will sustain their progress and helps them enjoy living with healthy habits the rest of their lives.

Chewing well is also essential for nutrient-optimizing absorption.

One of my mantras is that salad is the main dish. Research consistently shows that raw vegetables have the most powerful associations with the reduction of cancers of all types. I encourage people to not just eat a side salad or a small soup bowl, but a full, nine-inch serving bowl of salad every day for lunch. Chewing thoroughly, up to 30 chews of each bite will liquefy each mouthful. There are potent enzymes that are present in the cell walls of vegetables such as the myrosinase enzyme in cruciferous vegetables and the alliinase enzyme in onions and scallions. When plant cells are crushed through chewing, the enzymes are liberated and activated to form isothiocyanates. Chewing well also increases the formation of organosulfur compounds, sulfenic acid, and nitric oxide in the mouth. It's not just eating a large salad every day, but it's also making sure each mouthful is well-chewed before swallowing to maximize healing potential.

I advise that lunch is the most important meal, comprised of a big salad with a nut- or seed-based dressing, a bowl of vegetable and bean soup cooked with onions and mushrooms, and maybe a piece of fruit for dessert. Dinner typically consists of raw vegetables with hummus, salsa, guacamole, or other plant-based dip along with a cooked vegetable dish, such as blanched or steamed mixed vegetables with a bean or intact grain, or an Asian wok meal, making sure to include plenty of greens each day.

The Nutritarian diet is high in raw and cooked vegetables, well-cooked beans, soybeans, nuts, and seeds that keep the glycemic effect of the diet low, even when fruit is a part of a meal. Fruit, when eaten with the meal, does not have the negative glycemic effects compared to white rice, white potato, white bread, and other high-glycemic carbohydrates. Even whole wheat bread or whole wheat flour, depending on how finely it is ground, is unfavorably high-glycemic compared to beans, lentils, split peas, and chickpeas. In general, the diet should contain very little to no flour and instead include intact grains like quinoa, kamut, and steel cut oats. Studies with people who switch from white potato products to whole grains show their diabetic parameters improved by 30% because whole grains are not as glycemically unfavorable as white potato. However, when they swap whole grains to beans, there is an additional 30% improvement of the glycemic load, or a 60% improvement in the glycemic load over white potato.

If we score carbohydrate choices on a hierarchical scale of quality- peas, lentils, and beans contain more beneficial polyphenols, fiber, and resistant starch. They are also more slowly digestible carbohydrates than grains and potatoes. These factors are especially critical for a person prone to diabetes, heart disease, or who urgently needs to lose weight. This is because lower-glycemic carbohydrates are absorbed slowly over several hours, which also discourages eating between meals. Those with diabetes do not require as much insulin to keep their glucose low. Beans do not stimulate appetite sensors in the same way, enabling individuals to retain better control over the number of calories that they eat to lose or maintain a healthy weight.

Typically, a person may feel worse the first week or so after switching to a clean, healthful diet. Detoxification or withdrawal is commonly experienced when stopping addictive substances, and this is seen commonly when a person ends the consumption of unhealthful foods, and their body is excreting waste products. The body can even utilize the inflammatory response to aid in the removal of retained toxic wastes. We learned about this in medical school, in the first couple of weeks of pathology class. The book by Robins and Cotran, *The Pathological Basis of Disease*, if I remember correctly stated, "The inflammatory response is closely intertwined with the process of repair. Inflammation serves to wall off, oppose, and remove injurious agents in an attempt to heal and reconstitute damaged tissue."

The inflammatory response, so often misinterpreted as disease, most often represents the body's efforts to self-repair. When a person has an asthma attack, for example, the cells lining the lung become inflamed in their efforts to reduce or remove toxins. The symptoms are not our enemy, the cause of the toxicosis is the underlying offending agent. We can suppress the inflammation with steroids, but that just increases the depth and extent of the toxicosis as it restores normal breathing. The way to facilitate a complete recovery from asthma is with superior nutrition that can enable detoxification and a reduction of retained waste products; then the inhaled steroids can be successfully weaned over months. Over time, as patients follow a nutritious diet, with juicing and the conservative use of supplements, inflammation and toxicosis go down. They can then slowly tapered off steroids within a period of three to six months.

Likewise, we suppress headaches with Tylenol, narcotics, and ergotamines, but that just makes more severe and frequent headaches occur down the road, otherwise called rebound headaches. There is no magic; drugs are toxic, and they work because of their toxic effects. The whole intent of most medical interventions is to suppress the inflammatory response to reduce the symptoms or expression of disease. This is the opposite of restoring good health. Health is not the absence of symptoms, and a person is not healthy if it means needing to consume toxic drugs every day.

Autoimmune diseases are also distortions of the inflammatory response in which the body attacks itself, indicating a chronic state of toxicosis along with immune system derangement.

This is often caused by a combination of nutritional inadequacy and the buildup of inflammatory substances that our body is exposed to from exogenous environmental toxins or endogenously produced metabolic waste. With autoimmune diseases, we may not be able to wean patients off drugs until they have followed the diet for three months to avoid triggering an attack. At the start, I often prescribe juicing twice a day which helps rapidly elevate the carotenoids or antioxidants in the tissues, including the skin. I find that even when patients are eating carrots, beets, greens, kale, and berries, nutrient levels measured in the skin don't automatically increase. It can take months to get the nutrients in tissues to a level offering a necessary degree of protection. Patients might have to eat a healthy diet for six to nine months to have levels of nutrients in their tissues anywhere near healthy. Eating healthy works, but it takes time. Juicing can aid in delivery of results faster. Patients achieve concentrated levels of nutrients in their tissues at a much faster rate so that they can often be weaned from autoimmune drugs in three months rather than six or nine.

My recommended juice is usually 1/3 carrot and beet, 1/3 cruciferous vegetables (often bok choy), and the final 1/3 a combination of lettuce, celery, and cucumber (mostly lettuce since lettuce has the lowest levels of oxalic acid and the most gut-friendly substances). This therapeutic drink provides a high concentration of beneficial carotenoids and isothiocyanates in an easily consumable form to quickly increase their tissue nutrient levels. A typical glass is approximately nine ounces with about three ounces of each type of juice, twice a day. This juice is in addition to eating three Nutritarian meals a day with a big salad, berries, and seeds.

To keep Alpha Lipoic Acid (ALA) and other anti-inflammatory omega-3s high, I emphasize walnuts and seeds, plus a supplement containing vegan docosahexaenoic acid (DHA). DHA is a very important omega-3 fatty acid for brain health. To achieve an optimal anti-inflammatory omega-3 index above five generally requires the addition of a supplement. In some cases, especially with inflammatory bowel diseases like ulcerative colitis and Crohn's, fish oil may work better in providing a higher amount of eicosapentaenoic acid (EPA) than a vegan source of these omega-3s. EPA offers the most natural form of omega-3s. In the case of nutritional therapies for depression, I also use real fish oil for a greater amount of EPA. Although DHA might be more protective against dementia, studies indicate that patients who are acutely suffering from dementia or who have inflammatory bowel disease, respond better to a higher dose of EPA.

These concepts are the starting foundation of the Nutritarian program- a healthy plant-rich diet, chewed thoroughly, and removing pro-inflammatory foods from the diet. Processed foods, oils, and fried foods, are the worst contributors in the development of autoimmune diseases and inflammatory bowel disease, as well as allergies and asthma. The only dietary fats consumed should come from raw nuts and seeds, which can also be blended into salad dressings and dips.

With these changes, patients often feel significantly better even by the end of the first month. Based on how they are doing after two months, it's often possible to begin slowly weaning them off drugs, or in some cases, to stop them. Medications for diabetes and high blood pressure are weaned off as they are no longer needed, typically within the first month.

Note: for asthma patients, it's important never to stop a drug suddenly because it can create a flare. Patients should be brought down slowly on inhalers, switching to a weaker inhaled steroid, fewer puffs, or cutting the dose down from one brand to a weaker brand of inhaled steroid. When the patient is well and it's appropriate to stop the steroid completely, a few days of fasting may prevent the worsening of symptoms. Fasting has a powerful anti-inflammatory effect. It is generally not compatible for people on steroids for asthma but may sometimes be trialed at low doses as they are being weaned.

If patients are on oral steroids for autoimmune conditions, these drugs should be stopped for at least a month before considering any fasting. Sometimes, with inflammatory bowel disease or asthma, I will fast people for short three-to-four-day periods and repeat this every three to four weeks to accelerate their healing. I've even found that the repeated use of short fasting is better than long fasting that can deplete the patient nutritionally, making them emaciated, frail, and weak. It's better to maintain muscle mass and bone mass, and to keep them healthy, living their life, and utilizing shorter intervals of fasting to help mitigate the residual effects of inflammatory compounds in the body. The goal is to help patients build a new biochemical system to reverse their conditions. With a new biochemistry, the body can now recover from autoimmune conditions. Sadly, severe patients who have been on immunosuppressant drugs for decades or who have very advanced conditions may not respond as well as those with milder forms of autoimmune diseases that have not been on drugs as long.

If I could only catch people before they start chemotherapeutic drugs like Remicade and other dangerous drugs that cause cancer, it would be so much easier to get them well. When a person is first diagnosed with these diseases, if doctors would just start them on the right nutritional program, it would be so much more effective to enabling recoveries. Drugs complicate things, and over time, just make people sicker.

If every doctor managed disease with nutritional protocols, instead of prescription pads, then patients would be given choices that work. With our population getting older, there's a lot of desire not just to live healthier and longer but to maximize quality of life. Being healthy in our later years, so we can fully enjoy our life, is what makes healthy eating so valuable. Many of my friends from high school are dead, or are sick, or couch potatoes. They can't even enjoy life. I love being fully active - hiking, skiing, surfing, and playing tennis, volleyball, and pickleball. What good is living longer if you have no life? Living in a nursing home is not living.

People often say, "I'm sure you can live longer and have less disease by eating healthy, but I don't want to give up the things I enjoy. I would rather live a shorter life and eat the things I enjoy and enjoy my life more now while I'm young." But that's a myth. That's the food addiction part of the primitive brain talking. You're not giving up a pleasure in life by avoiding foods that are harming you. And your taste buds get more sensitive, adapting to like what you eat regularly. Healthful foods eventually taste just as good, if not better, than junk food. Eating in a self-destructive manner does not bring happiness. It brings tragedy and sadness to people's lives.

My patients are introduced to foods and incredibly delicious recipes that taste as good as anything you can get in a fine restaurant. The food we eat not only satisfies the senses but allows people to live and age well and avoid being sick in their later years, with the same agility, strength, and abilities they had when they were young.

Moderate caloric restriction in the context of micronutrient excellence is the secret to a long life.

Excess fat on the body speeds up our metabolism and accelerates aging. We have to modulate our calories and the type of foods we're eating to keep a minimum body fat percentage. At the same time we need to ensure high nutrient density in our tissues by consuming all of the nutrients that humans need. It's not difficult to do this when you're eating plenty of raw vegetables and greens, beans, and seeds. Not only will you feel satiated while eating all the foods you desire, but you will lose the need or desire to overeat. The volume of natural plant foods occupies space, triggers nutrient receptors and appetite receptors in the hypothalamus. Fast food, sweets, and oils, do the opposite, and induce overeating behavior.

For example, because of their resistant starch content all the calories in beans are not absorbed. Similarly, part of the calories of nuts are excreted into the toilet. You may feel like you ate 400 calories, and are satiated, but only 300 calories eventually get absorbed. Therefore, moderate caloric restriction achieves results just by choosing the right foods. We desire the right number of calories when we eat optimally. Notice that there are no overweight deer or squirrels or coyotes running around in the woods. There shouldn't be any overweight people either. People shouldn't have a roll of fat on their waist. Everyone can be naturally thin when they eat right.

Dietary excellence should be combined with exercise, so not only do we optimize phytochemical exposure, but total body exercise contributes to balancing the caloric needs of the body.

Total body exercise also amplifies longevity proteins, slowing the rate at which we age.

Remember, a moderately slowed metabolism means we age slower. The fallacy most people believe is that it is favorable to speed up their metabolic rate so that they can eat more food and not get fat, when the opposite is true.

We can age slower and live longer when we desire less calories, moderately slow the metabolic rate, and maintain good musculature with aging. This can all be achieved through an understanding of a Nutritarian diet and Lifestyle Medicine.

Chapter Nine

Neal D. Barnard MD – Diabetes, Hot Flashes, and Thyroid: Nutrition Interventions

Neal D. Barnard MD, is a clinical researcher, founding president of the Physicians Committee for Responsible Medicine (PCRM), and best-selling author. ↗pcrm.org

I would like to walk you through some new concepts in medicine. Most people think about health in a simple way. If I eat bad foods, they could cause some disease. I could gain weight, get high cholesterol, become diabetic, or something like that. What I'd like to suggest is that we think about the relationship between food and disease in a little bit more powerful way. Let's say, I eat food and that food affects my hormones in some way. Well, hormones affect everything in our body. And so, if we can control our hormones, we can change our weight. We can lose weight, and we can do all kinds of things that we'd really like to be doing, just by avoiding specific foods.

What are hormones, how do I control them; and how can I get them working in my favor? To answer, "What are hormones?" I could say, they are like a letter in the mail. They are made in one part of the body; for example, the thyroid is located at the base of the front of your neck. The thyroid hormone goes through the blood to the cells of your body giving them energy or insulin. From the pancreas, the hormone of insulin goes to the muscle cells to let sugar inside. This is the ideal mechanism. But sometimes our hormones go haywire. What I mean by this is, you're not getting enough letters in the mail. Sometimes the hormones just aren't being produced. Or even the complete opposite can happen, and your body can send out too many of these hormones. Your body can produce too few or too many hormones; either way it poses a big problem.

DIABETES

Let me show you how you can use food to get your body in balance and control the different hormonal functions. We'll start with insulin. As you know, insulin is the hormone influencing diabetes. It is made in the pancreas, goes through the blood to the muscle and liver cells, and acts like a key to let sugar into the cells for energy.

In 2003, the National Institutes of Health gave a grant to my research team to explore a healthy diet for diabetics. We wanted to know specifically if we could find an optimal diet to cure or prevent diabetes. The testing that we did was to evaluate a conventional diet versus a completely plant-based diet.

Let me describe the difference of these two types of diets. The conventional diet approach is what you'd expect to have recommended to you at a typical clinic- a reduction of calories and refined carbohydrates, and avoidance of bad oils and fats. But the new approach, the plant-based approach, allows for no animal product intake. This is a vegan diet. We minimize bad fats and use low glycemic index foods.

If that's a new term for you, white bread is an example of a high glycemic index food. High glycemic foods spike blood sugar. Relatively speaking, some bread, like pumpernickel, has a low glycemic index. Low glycemic carbohydrates offer a slow release. Beans, in general, are a high carb and starch food, but offer slow release. The lower the glycemic level of foods, the healthier they are. Here are some examples.

GLYCEMIC INDEX

Low (<55), High (70>)

HIGH	LOW
Muesli (80)	Grapefruit (25)
Baked potatoes (85)	Bran cereal (42)
Corn taco shell (97)	Cucumber (15)
White bread (100)	Lettuce (15)
Bagel (103)	Chickpeas (33)
Watermelon (72)	Lentils (41)
Pretzels (83)	Cherries (22)

Specifically, our testing tracked hemoglobin A1c. This is the index that we use for blood sugar measurement.

This improvement to health is with no medication, only dietary changes. And it's quite profound.

When we started seeing these results, we looked closely at our first patient in this study. He was on a vegan diet, lost 60 pounds, and was able to stop his diabetes medications. His high A1c dropped into the normal range. This was confirmation that his diabetes was gone. We are told in medical school that this is impossible. Now we see it all the time.

Let me explain to you how this diet works. And I can to show you what causes diabetes.

In the picture below is a purple oval representing a cell. Let's say it's a muscle cell in your body fueled by glucose, like its gasoline to the cells. The glucose needs to get into the cell to power it. But it can't get through the cell membrane, it just keeps bouncing off. We need a "key" to open the cell membrane for the glucose to pass through. What is preventing the glucose from getting into the cell? Doctors call it intramyocellular lipid- a buildup of fats from oils in chicken, beef, and fish.

With the insulin key, the glucose can get into the cell. When the insulin key is not working, the glucose can't pass through, and we call this insulin resistance.

What do we do in this case? One option is taking pharmaceuticals the rest of your life to force this action. This is the usual approach. Another approach would be changing the diet. A low-fat, vegan diet would prompt built-up fats to begin to break down and clear the openings.

And when that happens, the insulin sensitivity returns, and now the glucose can go out of the blood and into your cells where it belongs. You can see the reverse of diabetes as the hormone of insulin does its job.

ESTROGENS, HOT FLASHES, AND MENOPAUSE

Next, let's talk about estrogens, hot flashes, and menopause. Most women are familiar with hot flashes. You're sitting in a room, and suddenly you're burning up. What's going on? Its vasodilation. The blood vessels in your skin are opening. It is like somebody is opening a radiator and pouring the heat in.

Research in the 1980s showed that most women in Japan had no hot flashes. A small 15% reporting some mild symptoms. Since that time, with the typical Japanese diet changing from a rice-based to a meatier diet, hot flashes increased to 40% in the female population. What happened here?

The first theory was that Japanese women historically eat a lot of tofu and other soy products. And soybeans have isoflavones that not only reduce cancer risk but are also like a medicine against hot flashes. Over time Japanese women continued eating soy products and began experiencing hot flashes. So why did hot flashes become more common as time went on?

We suspected it was mostly due to their dietary changes with rice falling out of fashion. Grains, in general, are not less frequently consumed. The historical Japanese diet has been mainly replaced with more fish, dairy, meat, eggs, and fats. We believe these dietary changes are driving not only hot flashes but all kinds of other hormonal issues including breast cancer.

Next let's move from Japan to Mexico, and specifically Chiminea where many women still follow the traditional Mayan diet. This is another group of women with little to no reports of hot flashes. Yes, this group of people don't eat rice or soybeans. Their main grain and food source is corn, or maize. Their diet also consists of beans and vegetables. One of their traditional staple vegetables is called la Chaya. This important cultural, staple food is a hardy, perennial tree spinach providing large nutritious leaves.

Could this diet have something to do with the absence of hot flashes among this group of women? Our research team set out to explore this. Our study focused on "waves" or vasomotor systems. We took our study group of post-menopausal women and split them into two groups. Half of the women went into a Group A and made no dietary changes. The other half was put on a simple diet of plant-based foods. The plant-based diet contained no animal products, was low in fats, and included half a cup of cooked soybeans daily. This group also included daily vitamin B12 into their diets.

After the 12-week trial, we noted our observations:

Group A-Traditional Diet	Group B- Plant-based Diet
No weight loss	Weight loss- up to 8#s

| Slight drop in hot flashes | Reduced hot flashes (5 to1) |
| No significant changes | 84% drop in moderate to severe hot flashes |

Additional studies showed the diet group also had marked improvements in other areas including psychosocial symptoms. There was something about the simple combination of a plant-based, low-fat diet with some soybeans that acted like a very safe medication. I do need to add that our Group A showed some improvements, but we were unable to identify why. These are a few possibilities.

1) The study was done between September and December. The cooler weather could have had an impact.
2) Participants could have been making changes to their diet that went unrecognized by us.
3) Hot flashes sometimes diminish on their own.

When talking about soybeans in this content, let's address people's concerns on effects of soybean products to cancer risk. Many studies show that soybeans actually reduce cancer probability. One study posted by the US National Library of Medicine from National Institutes of Health research, in December of 2016, supports most findings, that soybean products reduce cancers rather than cause harm. [18]

> *Soy foods have long been recognized as sources of high-quality protein and healthful fat, but over the past 25 years these foods have been rigorously investigated for their role in chronic disease prevention and treatment. There is evidence, for example, that they reduce risk of coronary heart disease and breast and prostate cancer. In addition, soy alleviates hot flashes and may favorably affect renal function, alleviate*

---

[18] http://www.ncbi.nlm.nih.gov/pmc/articles/PMC5188409

depressive symptoms and improve skin health. Much of the focus on soy foods is because they are uniquely-rich sources of isoflavones. Isoflavones are classified as both phytoestrogens and selective estrogen receptor modulators.[i]

What we found was that women consuming the most soy products had a 29% reduced risk of developing breast cancer. But what if a woman has breast cancer already? If she avoids soy, her projected mortality increases. If she was to include soy products in her diet- milk, edamame, and tofu, she could cut her risk of dying from cancer by 25-30%. This is important because many people have been wondering about this. Somewhere along the way, a lot of people were told that soy would increase the risk of cancers in women. Extensive research shows quite the opposite. Soy products reduce the risk of cancer, and they reduce the risk of dying from cancer for those who have had it in the past.

THYROID

Let's talk next about the thyroid. The thyroid oversees your body's use of energy. It's a very modest organ; most people are unaware it is there. It's at the base of the front of your neck, and has the shape of a butterfly. It is a small but powerful and important organ. Its main function is producing a hormone. What is the importance of this hormone? It is extremely essential to the functioning of the whole body.

When your body doesn't produce enough of this hormone, you are said to be "hypothyroid" with symptoms impacting your whole body negatively, such as:

- The sense of "running on empty"
- The whole body feeling weakened
- Extreme sensitivity to cold
- A malfunctioning digestive track
- Weight gain

- Depression

The opposite can even happen. You can be "hyperthyroid." Hyperthyroid means you are producing too much thyroid hormone. Some of these symptoms are:

- Weight loss
- Rapid pulse
- Overactivity, feeling always revved up
- Nervousness
- Feeling always warm or hot, like you're overheating
- Sleep problems
- Skin and hair issues

What we know about the thyroid hormone thyroxine (T4) is that it needs iodine to function properly. The thyroid needs iodine to convert into T4, with the T4 being 65% iodine. The body doesn't need very much, 150 micrograms daily is all. Without this, there is hypothyroidism.

In 1924, the Morton Salt Company introduced iodized salt. This is the one with a little girl and the umbrella on the paper wrapper. This introduction very rapidly eliminated much of the iodine deficiency across the United States. And so, the thyroid was provided iodine that it needed. Today, people seem to be using more "modern" salts like sea salt, kosher salt, and Himalayan pink salt. While Himalayan and sea salt contains natural iodine, kosher salt does not. This has caused a large amount of the population to dip down into hypothyroidism again, along with all the bad press on salt being bad for us.

Another source of iodine besides salts is dairy, in a round-about-way. The dairy industry uses an iodine-laced disinfectant to clean the cow udders of encrusted milk, dirt, and mud. Some of these dribbles down through the milking tubes and into the milk. The dairy industry likes to say their products are a good source of iodine. This might be a source of iodine, but it certainly is not my favorite source.

The best source I think people should know about is sea vegetables. I grow up in North Dakota and never heard of foods like nori, wakame, or arame. What is this stuff? These are common foods found on a Japanese sushi bar. Nori is a dried edible seaweed, usually used as a vegetable wrapper, and is a great source of iodine. Wakame and arame are other forms of seaweeds.

Another good Japanese food full of iodine is miso soup. It provides a bounty of iodine as well as many other healthy nutrients. It is known to improve cardiovascular and digestive health. And another most delightful and fresh dish is a cucumber salad. These and other recipes can be found in my book *Your Body in Balance: The New Science of Food, Hormones, and Health.*

So that we don't think our thyroid health is only about getting enough iodine, let's look at some other issues involving the malfunctions.

Some people have antibodies to their thyroid glands. This is actually the main cause of hypo and hyperthyroidism in the United States. Let's walk through this.

Researchers have looked at whether foods could somehow trigger this. The Adventist Health Study, with more than 60,000 participants, found that people who are following vegan diets had a low prevalence of hypothyroidism. The people who did the worst were the lacto-ovo vegetarians. This is the group of non-meat-eating vegetarians who get protein from other dairy products.

When we look at the relationship between vegetarianism and thyroid imbalances, we see that vegans and vegetarians have the healthiest thyroid functions. Who seems to have the most thyroid malfunctions? It is the omnivores, those people consuming milk, meats, and eggs.

What we believe is happening is that the proteins in dairy and meat may trigger the release of antibodies that attack the thyroid. And if they attack the thyroid's ability to make the right hormone, you end up with hypothyroidism, diagnosed as Hashimoto's thyroiditis. If this attack causes the thyroid's ability to turn off, then you become hyperthyroid, or with a medical diagnosis of Graves' disease.

Let's walk though this together with a client named Nancy. Nancy was a 49-year-old accountant. She was hypothyroid since age 19. She was overweight, fatigued, and sensitive to cold. She was treated with thyroid supplementation, but she still didn't feel well. Her weight went up, her cholesterol went up, and both hit the same number, 265. She finally decided to change her diet. She went on a completely plant-based diet and her weight fell to 150. Her cholesterol dropped below 150, and her thyroid returned to normal. She no longer needed thyroid supplementation at all. And she feels terrific now. She noticed what a lot of people notice, that when you lose excess weight, your energy comes back, and your physiology improves. And with increased energy you can get involved with activities you had only dreamed off. In Nancy's case, she started running 5Ks.

A PLANT-BASED, HEALTHY DIET

So what is a healthy diet? A healthy diet is basically fruits, grains, vegetables, and legumes. The legume family includes beans, lentils, and peas. Small amounts of vitamin B12 are needed along with a plant-based diet for healthy nerves and blood. With a healthy plant-based diet you want to be sure you include some good vitamin B12, just a small amount, but daily.

If starting a vegan diet sounds a little daunting, let me show you how we do it in our clinic. We've used this with thousands of people and with much success.

A patient says, "I want to get rid of my diabetes" or "I'd like to lose weight" or whatever it is. I encourage them to take a week and look at what a vegan diet would mean for them, just check out the possibilities. I tell them to not think of it as starting a new diet but discovering new foods.

We start with a piece of paper to make a list. We brainstorm for ideas of foods they would enjoy. They develop their own list that might look something like this:

BREAKFAST	LUNCH
Oatmeal, cinnamon, raisins	Vegan pizza
Cereal with almond milk	Bean burrito
Barley with soymilk	Veggie burger

DINNER	SNACKS
Spaghetti	Fruit
Bean dishes	Carrot/Celery sticks
Veggie fajitas	Rice pudding
Rice	Hummus

We discuss that even eating out can offer good choices. Italian restaurants offer many different pasta and veggie dishes. Latin American and Mexican restaurants usually have a variety of bean and rice dishes. Chinese restaurant choices center around rice, vegetables, and tofu. Japanese meals offer edamame and different seaweed salads. Fast food is not the pinnacle of culinary art, but most places are now offering vegan options. After a few days of working on your list, you'll have it nailed down.

Once you have your list that you can use for grocery shopping you can then implement the diet for three weeks. A short time frame makes it doable. And with determination and a list in hand, you're ready to go. By this time, some things will begin to happen:

1) You will physically begin feeling better.
2) Your blood sugar level will improve.
3) You'll have increase energy.
4) Your mood and sleep should be improved.

Then you'll realizing you hadn't had chicken wings in three weeks, and you didn't miss it. Most people will also report in addition to discovering new foods, they are enjoying new books, movies, websites, and products in their life. People are encouraged to keep going on with their new diet and the new body they find themselves in.

To talk more about soy, what kind are we going to eat or drink? Which ones are better? And the same questions can go for olive oil. When we look at soy products, they all seem to reduce cancer risk, regardless of what kind of soy products we eat. However, if you find yourself with a choose of GMO (Genetically Modified Organism), which was developed for animal feed, avoid that. Find non-GMO products ideally, no matter what you eat.

If you are or were eating chicken, realize that most all chicken these days are raised on GMO soy and corn. If you're eating roast beef, same story. Finding non-GMO products for your diet is paramount to your health. By law, if the tofu package or the soy milk that you buy says organic, it cannot be GMO. I always recommend eating non-GMO foods.

And in my opinion, olive oil beats the heck out of chicken fat. If you look at any kind of oils or fats, they're always a mixture of bad and good fats. So, chicken fat could be up to 30% saturated fat, that's the one that raises your cholesterol. Olive oil is only about 14%, but for my money, I'd like to be at zero. So, I don't use olive oil at all although it's better than animal fats. If you're trying to lose weight, you might want to keep all fats and oils low, including nuts, seeds, and guacamole. There are some health benefits from nuts and seeds as they contain vitamin E, but they sure aren't helpful with losing weight. And if you're trying to lose weight or trying to tackle diabetes, you want to keep fats and oils low in your diet. I suggest going easy on the nuts and seeds at that point.

For those who are seriously interested in making dietary changes to a plant-based and healthy diet, I offer these steps.

1) Open your calendar and pick seven days.
   - Make a food list for this time-period.
   - Spend time looking for substitutes, like vegan bacon or sausage for your morning breakfast.
   - Try new foods.
   - Look for healthy options at restaurants.

2) Open your calendar and pick three weeks.
   - Make a food list for this time-period.
   - Determine to go all plant based.
   - Evaluate how you feel at the end of each week.

You will be amazed at all the wonderful results that a plant-based diet will bring to many areas of your life.

Chapter Ten

Ocean Robbins - The Science of Behavior Change (How to Influence People to Change Their Diets!)

Join bestselling author and Food Revolution leader, Ocean Robbins, to learn about the neuroscience of habit change; the root sources of human motivation; the right use of willpower; how to be a positive influence on the food choices of patients, loved ones, and family members; and what it's going to take to reverse the chronic disease epidemic in our lifetime.
↗ foodrevolution.org

We are certainly living in challenging times, to say the least, but also incredibly exciting times rich with opportunity. In no place, perhaps, is the opportunity more evident than in the arena of food. My name is Ocean Robbins, I founded the Food Revolution Network along with my dad John Robbins. He is a three-million-dollar bestselling author, social activist, and humanitarian.

I'll start with a little background of our story, move on a little bit to talk about the Food Revolution. And then we'll talk about how you can implement the program and practices into your own life.

First, a family story. My grandpa founded the Baskin Robbins ice cream company. My dad, John, grew up with an ice cream cone-shaped swimming pool in the backyard, and 31 flavors of ice cream in the freezer. He was groomed to one day run the family business. When he was in his early 20s, he was offered that chance, but he said no. He walked away from a path that was practically paved with gold and ice cream. We jokingly say in our family, "He followed his rocky road."

139

He then ended up moving with my mom to a little island off the coast of Canada, where they built a one-room log cabin and grew most of their food. They practiced yoga and meditation for several hours a day, and they named their son Ocean. That of course, would be me. They almost named me Kale, by the way, and that was way before kale was cool. But we did eat a lot of kale along with cabbage, carrots, and other veggies right from the garden.

When I was a little older, we moved to California. My dad researched the food industry in which he grew up and wound up writing a book called *Diet for a New America*, which came out in 1987. It inspired millions of people to look at their food choices as a chance to make a difference in the world. The media called him the "Rebel Without a Cone," and "The Prophet of Non-profit." Here was this would-be ice cream heir who walks away from immense wealth to pursue a path focused on health. The response was tremendous. All over the world, people were moved. And so, as I grew up in a family that was passionate and talking about food around the dinner table all the time, I kept seeing the impact that it was having on people's lives.

I saw the huge impact on Grandpa Irv, especially. My grandfather had lost his brother-in-law and business partner, Burt Baskin, to heart disease he was only 54 years old. And now, at the age of 69, in the late 1980s, my grandpa was facing his own serious heart issues. He had high blood pressure and blockages. He was also facing diabetes, obesity, and other weight related issues. His doctors told him that he didn't have long to live if he didn't make some big changes. They gave him a copy of my dad's book *Diet for a New America*. The amazing thing here is that my grandpa, who had manufactured and sold more ice cream than any human being who has ever lived, read the book, and made big changes. He ended up cutting out sugar and most processed foods.

He cut way down on his daily consumption, gave up ice cream and sugar, and lost a lot of weight. He reversed his diabetes and heart disease. He got off a lot of medications he had been told he would be taking for the rest of his life. His golf game improved seven strokes, and he lived 19 more healthy years.

We have seen in our family that when you eat the modern, industrialized diet, you get the modern industrialized diseases.

We have also seen that when you make a change, you can get tremendous results. Of course, my grandpa's story is not unique. We've seen this happen thousands of times and have received countless letters from people telling us how this message has changed their life and even saved their life in many cases.

When I was 16, I founded a non-profit with the objective of taking a healthy lifestyle message to my generation. It resulted in me working with young leaders in 65 countries for over two decades. As I traveled the globe, our program focused on youth leadership and empowerment. I saw the impact that diet had on people's health all around the world. I realized that my country, the United States, was the world example for exporting food processes. This involved producing and exporting Genetically Modified Organisms (GMOs) and pesticide containing foods. I also observed the United States methods of marketing and manufacturing processed food with companies like KFC, McDonalds, and even Baskin Robbins. These processes not only moved huge amounts of foods around the world, but also saw the expansion of waistlines and increases in health-related illnesses causing hospitalizations. Many were suffering with illnesses and diseases that were virtually unheard of in prior generations.

After 20 years of running this non-profit, I decided I needed to focus on food directly. I ended up joining with my dad and we launched "Food Revolution Network" in 2012. Since then, our mission has been a commitment to healthy, ethical, sustainable food for all. Those are big words, and the food revolution is a big concept. But I want to say how fundamentally important it is right now, to lay out the stakes of what is going on as well as what's ahead of us.

We live in a world where every day, human beings are fueling resource consumption, excessively raising and killing animals for meat, destroying forests around the globe, rendering topsoil useless, and poisoning water in our aquifers and water sources everywhere. Every day there is more carbon dioxide (CO_2) in the atmosphere and more pollutants in the environment. It doesn't take a rocket scientist to realize we are on a collision course with systemic environmental collapse. We have more and more people on this planet every day, and less and less natural resources, fewer fish in our oceans, and fewer nutrients in our soil. This cannot continue. If we can't grow food sustainably, then there will be no viable future for humanity.

The good news is, we can do something about it. Let's start with the most low-hanging fruit, which is eating lower on the food chain.

Right now, around the world, animal agriculture is responsible for over 70% of all agricultural land that humans are using. If just theoretically, the entire world went vegan tomorrow, which I'm not saying that's going to happen, but just hang out with me here for a second just to imagine this, we could immediately free up a land mass area equivalent to the United States, China, Australia, and the European Union combined. That much land is currently being used to graze cattle and other livestock, or to grow soy, corn, or other feed for animals. We have a terrible feed conversion ratio (FCR) with this system because it takes a lot of calories of input to create one calorie of flesh in an animal. The other portions of the ratio go to hoof, hide, bones, manure, body

142

heat, energy that the animal uses to move around, and gases that are coming out of the animals that are fueling climate change.

When we eat lower on the food chain, we free up this huge area of land which could go back to forests or other carbon sinks that could help to reverse climate change. It could also be used for solar and wind farms, or to grow food sustainably for the expanding human population. We need to be thinking of future generations. There are so many things we could do with that land that is not available to us right now. Instead, we're clear-cutting the tropical rainforest right now for grazing cattle. This should seem insane to any human being who wants their kids, grandkids, and future generations to have a sustainable future.

At the same time, we're using up water sources around the world. I live in California. There is currently a drought here, and in much of the United States. All over the world, water is almost as valuable as fuel because in so many places the aquafers are being depleted. We're using up water that's been stored up over millennia. Again, I want to remind you, we can do something about this. We can have a positive impact by eating lower on the food chain. This helps free up land and water because it would save all the irrigation water going to the croplands and the feeding of livestock. Did you know, it takes about 2000 gallons of water to produce one pound of feedlot beef in the United States today? That's a lot of water. That means you could stack a pile of one-gallon jugs of water almost half a mile high with the water you would save by not eating one pound of beef. This is tremendous, right? It's leverage. And it's not just the planet that's at stake. It's also our own lives.

In 2019, The Institute of Health Metrics and Evaluation, produced a report *Global Burden of Disease.* [19]

---

[19] https://www.healthdata.org/gbd/2019

This report is an extensive global study of hundreds of researchers reporting the major causes of death and disability around the world. They look at lifestyle and environmental factors. These researchers concluded that the modern diet is the central driving force behind 672,000 deaths in the United States and more than 11 million worldwide annually. When you look at this fact, we can see that year after year our diet fuels epidemic rates of:

- Heart disease -The leading cause of death on the planet
- Diabetes
- Alzheimer's
- Obesity

More than half of the U.S. population over the age of 85 have Alzheimer's.

But it doesn't have to be that way. We now know that most lifestyle illness can be prevented, and much of it can even be reversed with diet and lifestyle choices.

When I say diet and lifestyle, I mean, eat less sugar and processed junk, eat fewer animal products especially from factory farms, eat more whole plant foods, and source consciously for more organic, fair trade, non-GMO, natural real foods, local foods; and with fewer pesticides, hormones, antibiotics, saturated fat, and more phytonutrients. That's the bottom line.

Now, I would like to ask you a question. With all that we know, why aren't we eating differently? I think it was Yoda who said to Luke in one of the Star Wars movies, "There is no try, there is just DO." So why don't we just DO it? I mean, it's not like we don't know that we need to eat more vegetables. It's not like we don't know that sugar is bad for us. But we're still eating gobs of sugar. We're still digging our graves and destroying the planet with our knives and forks. We know this as a society and as individuals.

Here's the thing, habits can be hard to change. They're deeply ingrained in each of us. Food is so intimate, and so personal. What you eat becomes you, and it's connected to your family, your history, your culture, and your sense of identity as a human. Quite frankly, your microbiome has been forged around the foods that are familiar to you. Even the bacteria in your gut are the bacteria that like the foods that you're used to feeding them. They're sending signals saying, "Give me more of that." Your body loves what's familiar, and we tend to be creatures of habit. Most of the time we don't do things because we give much thought to it, we do things on autopilot. Even the way that we speak is forged out of habits that were formed before we even learned to talked. We learned from watching our parents communicate. And that's why we speak the language we do. That's why a lot of the ways that we think are ancestral because things get passed down without anyone even being aware of it.

Food is one of the areas where what you think you like or what you're drawn to is what's familiar and easy. Your path of least resistance is what you've always done. But here's the problem with that. If we keep doing what we've always done, we're going to get more and more of the same equal toxic food culture, equal suffering and misery, chronic diseases, and the likelihood of fueling a devastating environmental collapse. Therefore, it is time for us to form new habits.

Here's the problem with that. A lot of people don't realize that willpower does not shape their destiny. It's habits that shape destiny. It's what you do day in and day out, when you're on autopilot, whether you're thinking about it or not, whether you're trying or not; all this fuels who you become and where you end up. If you step out of the paradigm, you can change course, you can get on a new path, and suddenly you're seeing a whole new landscape. You'll find it's the steps you take one after the other that get you to a new place.

So right now, wherever you are in your journey, I want to invite you to ask yourself, are you on a path that leads you where you want to go? And if you're not, this might be a moment to reorient, realign, and recognize that food can be medicine. Food can be an act of integrity. Food can represent your love for yourself and your planet. And when you put all this together, you recognize the incredible power you have with every bite that you take when you claim that power wisely, consciously, and intentionally. You can change your life, and you can change the world. But it starts with habits. The right use of willpower is to form new habits, and then let them get deeper and deeper engrained. Then the willpower kicks as a new habit to keep you on your path.

The best time to repair a roof is when the sun is shining; you don't do it when it's pouring down rain.

The best time to change a bad habit isn't when you're starving or exhausted. The best time is to start is at the beginning of a week, on a weekend, or when life offers you a little extra time.

Here are some tips for helping you create sustainable habit change.

1) Shop in bulk and cook in quantity. Make friends with leftovers to avoid going to the store every day.
2) Plan and make friends with the bold staples in your kitchen.
3) Cook up a pot of legumes once or twice a week. They keep well and they pair with a lot of other foods. Lentils, beans, split peas, all are good daily staples.

4) Keep some cooked grains in the fridge. Quinoa, amaranth, millet, buckwheat, and other grains are all healthy staples to have handy for breakfast, lunch, or dinner.
5) Keep a stock of fresh vegetables on hand. They provide a very versatile food group.
6) Plant a garden. There is no better place to get fresh vegetables from than your own back yard.
7) Cooked vegetables are handy and adaptable to a lot of dishes. They mix and match well with other veggies and grains, or can easily be made into casseroles.
8) Add steamed vegetables to anything whether you're making pasta, a casserole, even oatmeal. Sounds crazy? Yes!

My favorite breakfast is a savory meal and I cook it in quantity. I cook enough for four breakfasts at a time, and I keep them in little metal containers in the fridge. I then have them ready to go, bust them out each morning, and I've got my breakfast. Very easy to warm and eat.

My most favorite breakfast is savory oatmeal. I make oatmeal in an instant pot the night before I want it. I cook it with unsweetened soy milk, chopped onions and garlic, some veggies, and soy sauce, along with some olive oil, cayenne pepper, and other spices. After it's cooked, I mix in some seeds, like pumpkin seeds or sunflower seeds. I also add ground chia meal or seeds, and nutritional yeast. Stir it all up. And I'll tell you what, it's pretty delicious. I make enough for four days in a row and it's ready to go. Bam! Breakfast is handled.

My leftovers from dinner are used for lunch the next day. Because I get going early in the day and I want to move through my day quickly, I don't want to spend the morning in the kitchen. Personally, the evening is a better time for me to do my planning and meal prep. Here are some tips that I've found help make my meal planning more efficient. Hopefully you can find some of these helpful to you.

1) Make friends with leftovers, cutting out on wasting food.
2) Weekly clean out your frig, make a big pot of soup or a stew. You can freeze leftovers and have meals ready to go.
3) Make extras to freeze for yourself and to share with others.
4) Get a co-op going at work where everybody brings health foods for a potluck once a week.
5) If you have a small group of five people, each can pick a day of the week to bring in lunch for everyone. Then each one cooks five meals for one day, but all five people get five different meals.

The bottom line with all of this is finding out what works for you. I'm sharing some tips and ideas. They might work for you, they might not. Or maybe you hate the idea of savory oatmeal. That's fine. I'm just telling you what I love to do to maybe spark some ideas. What I am saying is that you've got to dedicate yourself to finding ways to get on the path that helps you succeed and thrive. Pay attention, be a student, get curious about what works.

Another big tip, by the way, is to clear out your kitchen of all the bad stuff. It's a lot easier to not have late-night cookie binges if there aren't cookies sitting in your cupboard. Clear away the foods that you don't want to be eating. A lot of people who are getting on the healthy eating path will get rid of all kinds of food. You can give it away to people who will be buy it anyway. Or send it off to the compost pile if you prefer. Then choose to focus your buying habits on the healthy foods that help you thrive. The best way to not eat junk food is to not buy junk food. It can be as simple as that.

Here are some additional thoughts and tips to help you get off to a solid start.

1) Find some good, healthy recipes that you're going to enjoy.
2) Don't beat yourself up if you fall off the horse. Get back up and try again.
3) Hold yourself in a lot of love every step of the way.
4) Keep moving forward, keep making progress.
5) Remember, it's what you do day-to-day that shapes your destiny.
6) If you slip occasionally, remember it's what you do 95% of the time that matters most.

Next, I'd like to share some words with you about hope. We live in a world in which a lot of people feel despair right now about the state of the planet, about their personal issues and problems, politics, things that just feel so broken and dysfunctional. It is easy to understand and feel the hopelessness sometimes. But I live with a lot of hope in my heart, and I want to tell you why. To me, hope is not so much of a noun as a verb. It doesn't come from calculating on the sidelines how things are going to go out there in the world; it comes from the actions we take and the choices we make personally. I know for a fact that we all have immense power to redirect the course of our lives as well as the world, into healthier directions.

The food revolution is alive and well. I am privileged to be a part of a movement that is changing the course of history. Every day there are more people choosing organically grown food. Every day there are more people switching over to plant-based diets, and the number of people who identify as vegan has quadrupled in the U.S. in the last decade. The number of farmer's markets and community-supported agriculture programs are skyrocketing. Interest in natural, healthy foods is increasing rapidly. The number of big food corporations that are starting to take an interest in natural foods is growing too because consumers are demanding it. They are fed up, we are fed up, with the status quo and are hungry for change.

Food and restaurant industries are finally starting to shift. Even government policies are getting rattled. Lifestyle Medicine advocates for produce prescriptions with doctors prescribing fruits and vegetables instead of or as well as drugs and surgeries. We're advocating for Double Up Bucks, where food aid programs help the poor with programs like the "Supplemental Nutrition Assistance Program" in the United States.

Many countries have a similar program to encourage an uptake of fruits and vegetables. We want to help low-income communities and families who are struggling, to have access to healthy and sustainable food. This is our mission, this our vision, these are our values, and we're getting traction. We are changing the world.

Some people talk about the pleasure of doughnuts or ice cream. And there's no doubt those are pleasurable. I think that 42% of people say that food is their number one pleasure in life. But here's the thing, even your taste buds are impacted by how you eat. By the age of 70, most people have lost half their taste buds. So even the pleasure of food drops over time. If you think back to childhood, you're like, "I remember how good things tasted." Well, partly you may be having a different experience now. But the truth is, the taste buds are connected to your cardiovascular health. When your body has the proper nutrients, it improves blood flow. With the proper blood flow, you have more capacity for pleasure in every cell of your body, including your taste buds. I'm a big fan of healthy pleasures that come from healthy food. And you can have so much more pleasure in your life when you're radically alive, full of joy, and your life feels complete.

In the health industry we find experts that will say just about anything. We find experts telling us we need to drink more, we need to drink less, we need to do intermittent fasting, or that we need to eat small portions throughout the day. We can find experts telling us that coconut and saturated fat are wonderful, and we can find experts telling us that they're very bad for our health. We can find experts saying of course, that vegetables are great, and we can even find "experts" nowadays, I put experts in quotes, telling us that we should be eating the carnivore diet and eating nothing but meat. Here's the thing. At the end of the day, I look to what the preponderance of studies tells us. And anytime somebody is like, what if everything you thought you knew about nutrition was wrong? I'm like, get out of town — because the human body hasn't radically changed.

There's not some bright new epiphany that is suddenly going to turn everything on its head when we have tens of thousands of studies published in peer-reviewed journals that give us a whole lot of insight. And that insight is super clear overall. Yes, there are nuances. Yes, there are new things we could learn. And yes, there are ways to hack the system and cheat the body, and even trick us or scare us into certain types of diets. Bottom line is, you want to base your diet around real "whole foods," mostly plants. Michael Pollan said it perfectly when he stated, "Eat food, as in real food, not processed junk, mostly plants, not too much." Basic and simple.

Follow the experts that you trust and keep leaning into their wisdom. I look to people like Dr. Joel Fuhrman, and Dr. Michael Greger. These are examples of trustworthy mentors and sources of good information.

We have over a thousand articles on our website now, with lots of helpful topics and resources. You can search and find trustworthy people. You will see they are well studied and credible. They are not just out to make a buck off some new fad diet. Listen, read, and see what they have to say. I offer you good sources to help you cut through the confusion. Confusion breeds apathy and apathy breeds status quo, and the status quo is what is killing us. We need to move forward. There are so many half-truths and partial truths out there. We need a finely tuned BS meter to quickly cut through it all. Learn to not believe everything you hear but to be drawn to those who can really help make a positive impact on your overall and long-term health.

Research studies are always interesting. You can look at them from different angles. Many people do and they spin them in different ways. Remember that the overwhelming body of evidence tells us that everyone does best by eating more vegetables, fruits, and whole plant foods.

Whole grains are good for us too. They're associated with lower rates of Alzheimer's, cardiovascular disease, and cancer. Legumes are good for us also. All the people in the blue zones, where people live the longest and healthiest lives, have a diet centered around legumes.

We also know that eating processed foods is not healthy for anyone. As far as animal products, most studies tell us that less is better. I know everyone's bodies and cells are different, but there are general health practices that we know are across-the-board best for everyone.

Some people do fabulously on a strictly vegan diet. Many vegans and vegetarians need to pay attention to getting enough omega-three fatty acids, especially DHA and EPA, and also supplementing with a few other nutrients like- vitamin K2, B12, and in some cases- zinc, selenium, or magnesium.

152

I don't believe protein should be the concern that it is made out to be. Most people, I believe, get more than they need rather than not enough. If you're vegetarian or vegan, it's good to make sure you are getting enough legumes and basic protein sources in your diet. But if you eat a diversity of whole plant foods, you're probably going to do just fine with all the required micro and macronutrients that your body needs. If you eat a highly processed diet or eat a lot of fats, this will definitely have a negative impact on your overall health.

Wherever you are on your journey, take a moment to:

- Look at your current health situation.
- Make a list of your health challenges.
- Write down any fears you are facing along with these challenges.
- Look at your lifestyle today?
- Decide what would you like your lifestyle to look like moving forward?
- Envision where you want to be when you are 70, 80, 90, and 100.
- Envision how you want to feel when you are 70, 80, 90, and 100.
- Ask yourself what you can change going forward?
  - Pain and suffering?
  - Visions and dreams?
  - Do you have longings for a different and brighter future?
- Ask yourself what steps you can take to connect to the big "why?"
  - How can you align to your "why" right now?
- Make a list of some steps you can take to align your life choices more fully with your visions and dreams, and what you really want your life to look and feel like.

153

- Make it happen.

George Bernard Shaw is quoted as saying;

> *"This is the true joy in life, to be used for a purpose recognized by yourself as a mighty one. Being a force of nature instead of a feverish, selfish little clod of ailments and grievances, complaining that the world will not devote itself to making you happy."*

> *"I am of the opinion that my life belongs to the whole community and as long as I live, it is my privilege to do for it whatever I can."*

> *"Life is no brief candle to me. It is a sort of splendid torch which I have got a hold of for the moment, and I want to make it burn as brightly as possible before handing it on to future generations."*

I want to thank you for burning your candle or your torch as brightly as you can and for being a part of the revolution in whatever ways you can.

Remember that every bite you take and every dollar you spend on food is a vote.

It is your vote for the health you want for yourself and the future. Together, let's make it a good one.

Chapter Eleven

Johannes R. Fisslinger MA, LPHCS - How to Prescribe Lifestyle *Medicine in 3 Minutes: Without Changing Your Workflow or Increasing Expenses*

Johannes is the founder of Lifestyle Prescriptions® University, HealthiWealthi™ RXHEAL Coach Platform & Ecosystem, author of "The 6-Root-Causes of All Symptoms, and the driving force behind the "Prescribing Lifestyle Medicine" and "Lifestyle Prescriptions®" movement. ↗ lifestyleprescriptions.tv

Does it happen to you too sometimes, that you have an idea or a thought popping into your head and you wonder what is this all about? This thought just bugs you, and it seems to come back again and again. What does it mean? What does it tell me? Do I need to do something about that?

This happened to me in 2013 when this whole idea of lifestyle prescriptions came into my head, popping in while I took a shower, or whenever I was meditating. That idea was harassing me. I thought it's an interesting concept. I mean, we've been writing different forms of prescriptions for decades or centuries, but nobody has thought about writing habit-improving Lifestyle Prescriptions®.

A few months later, the thought came back again, and I felt now I really need to dive into this topic. I googled related terms and could only find green prescriptions which were about nature, having a walk and similar activities.

Like so many times in my life, when these innovative ideas arose inside of me, I waited for a while until I realized that nobody else is going to do it. So I have to.

After outlining a structure how to use Lifestyle Prescriptions® in medicine I realized that the implementation is going to be the big issue.

Again, this is very much for health professionals, but also for health lovers, for anyone who is interested in healthy living.

Healthcare is really complicated, complex with special interest not wanting to change the status quo. The idea that healthcare professionals and patients alike just accept the Lifestyle Prescriptions® innovation is an illusion. I'm very realistic about that. Change is hard.

If doctors have a successful and profitable practice why would they integrate something that benefits patients but adds more work with no reimbursement or added revenue? If someone with a quick-me-fix-mentality is sick it's so much easier to pop a few pills and feel better instead of addressing the root-causes and improving their diet, exercise more, manage psychosocial and life stress better, and improve love and support in their life.

Forget about it! It's too complicated.

But what if it is possible to prescribe lifestyle medicine in just three minutes, without even changing (and I'm talking to health professionals now) your workflow, or hiring expensive staff?

What if we remove the complications, make it so easy that integrating Lifestyle Prescriptions® is a no-brainer?

When we added the concept of micro-habits, then the implementation of writing Lifestyle Prescriptions® completely changed. Because suddenly it was equally easy for clients and patients to improve their lifestyle habits without being overwhelmed or believing it's difficult, hard and lots of will-power is needed. In fact, no will-power is required by improve one tiny small habit at a time. With repetition comes automation and like our smartphone app it happens without us noticing it.[20]

Micro-habits are tiny, little steps that I can do as an individual.

We change a tiny step or small procedure, add or remove something that has a powerful effect on how we live or perceive life. The 20/80 rule, or even the 1 to 80 rule applies to micro-habits, where we change something small, which then grows into something really big. That's the idea.

Just think about it for a second, if every doctor in the country and worldwide would prescribe lifestyle medicine. If every doctor in the world has two prescription pads, one Rx pad for managing and treating diseases, and another for writing Lifestyle Prescriptions® to address the root-causes and help clients stop and reverse chronic symptoms.

I'd like you to visualize you visiting your doctor and to your surprise he is offers you a choice and says, "Do you want to manage the symptoms or do you want to address the root-causes of the chronic symptoms by using evidence-based Lifestyle Medicine protocols?"

WOW.

I'd like you to visualize this and make it large and big. Because next time you go to a health professional, what do you ask? Whenever you go to your next doctor's office visit, you say in a confident way to your doctor:

"Do you offer lifestyle medicine for my condition?"

"Do you prescribe lifestyle medicine?"

---

[20] Tiny Habits: BJ Fogg Standford University, www.tinyhabits.com

This is powerful. If you and 10,000s of others ask these questions then we're going to create a movement that will make Lifestyle Medicine and Health Coaching accessible to everyone.

Now, if you're a health professional, you might say, I don't have time to train and it's expensive. I just can't do this, I can't think about it, just stop. Stop.

Ask yourself if this is really true. Really?

Dr. Shirzai said, *"We always have three minutes for our patients, right? For every client."* And if a client gets the option, a choice, and wants to go the lifestyle medicine preventive route, then shouldn't we support them?

Naturally and just to be very clear, we're not talking about an emergency. We're not talking about a situation where we need to manage a client's symptoms.

We're talking about stopping or reducing chronic symptoms and there is always time and a way to write a Lifestyle Prescription® which could be as simple and beneficial as referring a patient to a certified health coach.

Again, it takes just a few minutes and asking a few questions to write that Lifestyle Prescription® for your clients; is rather easy to do. It does not require years of training; it requires a willingness to start that process. Once you start doing it, you will see that it's a lot easier than you thought.

Let's dive into and explore the world of prescriptions.

CLIENT BENEFITS	PRACTITIONER BENEFITS
Offers choices	A sense of pride
Feeling of self-empowerment	Less burnout
Long-term health solutions	Client respect and appreciation

When introducing people to Lifestyle Medicine and Lifestyle Prescriptions® we should assume most of the general populace in the world will not be familiar with this term. We can explain it in comparison with modern medicine.

MODERN MEDICINE	LIFESTYLE MEDICINE
Manages disease	Prevents, stop & reverse symptoms
Often unwanted side effects & complications	Many positive, health-enhancing side effects
Expensive	Low-cost, for all ages
	Improves vitality, immunity
	Activates auto-regulation, homeostasis and self-healing
	Addresses all root-causes including body-mind

Since we started to use the term Lifestyle Prescriptions® and implemented it into our Lifestyle Prescriptions® University Training programs, may other terms have been used including lifestyle medicine prescriptions, prescribing lifestyle medicine, social or nature prescribing which are wonderful but also distinctively different from Lifestyle Prescriptions®.

PRESCRIBING LIFESTYLE MEDICINE

Let me explain the differences starting with lifestyle medicine prescriptions, prescribing lifestyle medicine

We have found that many people take a "wait and see approach" to their personal health issues. Then when the symptoms are severe, they want immediate results. The body doesn't work that way.

The moment you have any symptom at all is the best time to pay attention to it. The first step to improving our health is awareness and the recognition that symptoms are signs and signals we need to pay attention to.

Lifestyle medicine prescriptions or prescribing lifestyle medicine relates typically to addressing chronic symptoms by improving our lifestyle habits based on the four pillars of Lifestyle Medicine as defined by Dr. Dean Ornish, considered to be the father of lifestyle medicine.

These four pillars of Lifestyle Medicine are:

- Nutrition
- Fitness or exercise
- Stress management
- Love and support

There are many ways to integrate this four-pillar approach with clients. One is prescribing Lifestyle Medicine.

There are many different types of diets that we can look at including- paleo, veganism, vegetarianism, raw foods, keto, the Mediterranean diet, and the list goes on and on. What's important to move towards a clean plant-based nutrition that includes less toxic, chemical or processed foods and is high in high quality nutritious foods.

There are many avenues to fitness and exercise including tennis, running, and walking. I personally play tennis and run. One of my personal Lifestyle Prescriptions® currently is running 15 minutes each morning. I have never been a morning runner before in my life but am really enjoying it.

Stress management techniques include deep breathing exercises, music, yoga, meditation, group therapy, counseling, and prayer. There is a plethora of self-help guides online just doing a simple search.

The last of the four pillars - love and support, are as important as the other areas. It includes self-love and self-care as well as the love and support one can feel with others. This also involved a social support system that can make or break some people emotionally.

All of these areas are considered important and integral to each Lifestyle Medicine aspects of health and wellbeing. Learning how to incorporate each area into our lives is essential.

Change can be difficult but with a guide and a coach it's going to be a lot easier. When you design your new habit, we suggest following the SMART principle and make it as specific, as attainable, measurable as possible.

S	SPECIFIC	DIRECT AND DETAILED
M	MEASURABLE	QUANTIFIABLE
A	ATTAINABLE	REALISTIC
R	RELEVANT	ALIGNS WITH GOALS
T	TIME-BASED	HAS A DEADLINE

Non-smart goals are:

- "I stop drinking sugary drinks."
- "I will eat better."
- "I go out in nature more often."
- "I am going to cut down on chocolate.
- "Relax as much as you can."

On the contrary, the following SMART micro-habits provide very clear instructions and guidance which will increase compliance.

- "I substitute sugary drinks with water for the next 7 days."
  "I increase my vegetable intake by 20% daily for 7 days."
- "I go for a 5-minute walk right after I return home from work for the next 7 days."
- "Whenever I desire chocolate, I eat an apple or banana."
- "I meditate for 10 minutes daily right after I brush my teeth for the next 30 days."

SMART goal setting is an approach that can be applied to any area of life and is very helpful when applying to lifestyle changes.

When working with clients and patients, we look for feedback.

We ask questions like, "Is that something you feel you can do?" Their physiology (voice, body or eye movements, breathing pattern) will provide clue to you of how they are feeling about what you asked. A "Yes, sure I do it." Does not mean they are motivated, committed, or know exactly why and how to perform that new habit.

Writing a Lifestyle Prescription® that works is mostly about motivation, having a highly emotional reason and intention that drives us into action.

The new habit must be agreeable with them and also realistic. If they say they can change their diets within one day, that's unrealistic. So, make only realistic goals with them.

It also must be time-based, where you as their doctor or healthcare provider agree on a Lifestyle Prescriptions®, then together "clunk it down." This means working together to bring something big to a small micro habit.

Here is some dialogue you could have with a client.

1. Are you willing to look at a small micro habit, to help change your health and wellbeing that is specific,

measurable, important and you absolutely know you can and will do?

2. What could that micro-habit be?
3. Why would you want to make that change?
4. How would you benefit from making that change?
5. Will you find pleasure in making this change?

See what answers your patients come up with. Do they want to be healthier to spend time with their grandchildren? Or maybe they just want to grow old with a keen and funny mind like Bernie Siegel? Determining the "why" of making a change is very important and will radically improve compliance.

You've determined the "why" with them. Next is the "how." When people don't know how to make changes it is nearly impossible for change to occur. Stepping them through a lifestyle change needs to be very specific. So back up the SMART with specific steps "how" to make this important change happen. With your client, state a change; then ask them:

1. Is this something you want to do?
2. Is this something you think you can do?
3. Is it Specific?
4. Is it Measurable?
5. Is it Attainable?
6. Is it Relevant?
7. Is it Time-based?

The next phase as the doctor or practitioner is to reframe and realign the change or goal. Cognitive reframing is changing the way we look at things. Wayne Dyer, bestselling motivational author summed up reframing in his book *Change Your Thoughts, Change Your Life*.

It is seeing the same thing, but differently.

If changing a habit seems difficult and doesn't give good warm-fuzzies, what would change? What could change? Asking how your client feels about the new habit is important to the feeling behind it, and the likelihood of success.

For example, when I started taking my daughter to school, I notice how nice and sunny it was getting outside in the morning. I started stretching, and it felt good. Then I thought of running a little and noticed how nice it felt. The next time I did this, it didn't feel like a big change but just a little micro habit. I started doing it every day for just ten minutes at the beginning. It didn't seem to take any willpower at all once it felt automatic. Then I started going further and further.

It's like when your computer pops up with a notification. Do you immediately respond? Not usually. You first want to know the benefits to you. Then if you see the benefits, you can schedule it on your time. This is similar to a smart automation in our unconscious mind. Since our brain and biology are linked, once there is good automation, it can run itself. Our body will perform out of automation and not by force to our willpower.

Another good thing about micro habits is that they provide a continuum of wins for the client.

If, for example, they don't drink soda today, that's a win. Then when they don't drink it the next day, it's another win. Then after a week, it is yet another win. Each step along the way they feel pride in their accomplishments.

Keep in touch with your clients and celebrate their accomplishments. This can be very motivational to them. They feel very special is even just getting an email from you.

The next time you meet, you can review the new habit with the client, and then set out together the next step. Are they ready to extend and deepen the new habit? Or are they ready to move forward and add another micro habit?

There are times when it is necessary to make more than just micro-habit changes. There are people with major health issues that need to make big changes starting out. Doctor Ornish says of this, *"The more comprehensive the lifestyle changes are, the more powerful and quickly the effects can be."*

Easier said than done though, I know.

LIFESTYLE PRESCRIPTIONS®

Lifestyle Prescriptions® takes the prescribing Lifestyle Medicine principles several steps further by adding Organ-Mind-Brain Anatomy™ into the mix.

Consider Organ-Mind-Brain Anatomy™ as an evolution to Anatomy. Without Anatomy medicine as we know it would not be possible. Without Organ-Mind-Brain Anatomy™ integrative, holistic or lifestyle medicine lacks a unifying foundation in terms of root-cause diagnostics or analysis.

The reality is that the mechanical-only model of the human body is totally outdated because we know that trauma, stress, perceptions, emotions, and limiting beliefs have a tremendous impact on every part of our body.

Organ-Mind-Brain Anatomy™ clearly defines which specific stress, emotions, beliefs/thoughts and lifestyle habits affect specific organ tissue which allows a trained Lifestyle Prescriptions® Practitioner to be very, very specific in what we call Root-Cause Analysis and in providing personalized and laser-sharp micro-habits that address one specific organ tissue symptom.

Please refer to the chapter Organ-Mind-Brain Anatomy™, the 6 Root-Causes and the Art and Science of Self-Healing for a more detailed explanation.

An integral part of Lifestyle Prescriptions® is realizing the importance of psychosocial stress because the reality is if I am absolutely in rage, stress hormones are high and all I can think about is how to survive by fighting my "perceived or real enemy" then what I eat, how I sleep, or how well I exercise becomes absolutely secondary. My life is focused around solving this "conflictive-stress loaded" situation. Once solved, the natural cycle of repair, regeneration and auto-regulation kicks in and at that point my thoughts and actions will refocus to eating better, exercising more, managing our day-to-day stress better, and increasing love and support.

"Initially described as resulting from a onetime severe traumatic incident, PTSD (Post-Traumatic-Stress-Disorder) has now been shown to be triggered by chronic multiple traumas as well." [21]

Science has demonstrated that re-experiencing of the traumatic event, avoidance of stimuli associated with the trauma, and symptoms of increased arousal will prolong PTSD/

What we also noticed is that "small" stress trigger that often appear not important can trigger us into psychosocial stress with increased hormone levels, sympathetic stress symptoms, high emotional arousal and conflict-active thoughts.

Psychosocial stress in general is relevant and one part of the six-root-cause wheel, but a very important one.

---

[21] https://www.ncbi.nlm.nih.gov/pmc/articles/PMC3181584/

What makes Organ-Mind-Brain Anatomy™ so unique is that we can assign different types of psychosocial stress to specific organ tissue.

In our empirical studies and practice us over three decades it became clear that stress is not generic affecting us but actually organ tissue specific.

For example, territorial type of anger like fighting with a competitor (real or perceived) often affects the stomach mucosa with ulceration increasing during the stress phase.

A loss of visual touch like our favorite child is leaving for college or our beloved husband died correlates with the conjunctiva being affected with inflammation of the skin layer during the regeneration phase.

Or a sense of no-low self-value, feelings of not being strong or good enough or not being able to withstand pressure affect the skeletal structure.

Just imagine if there would be a "map" of how organ, mind, brain interact in a specific way that is not random? Using Organ-Mind-Brain Anatomy™ allows us to decode our body's self-healing mechanisms and be very specific with writing Lifestyle Prescriptions®.

Helping clients become aware that symptoms are not random or meaningless and that every organ tissue in their body has a specific psychosocial stress connection is deeply impactful. Because suddenly, we get answers to the WHY - Why is this happening to me?

Here's an example of a client with chronic eczema on the right inside arm.

His doctor prescribed medicines and his naturopath prescribed herbs to treat the symptom.

Using the Lifestyle Prescriptions® Root-Cause Analysis process we would first ask a few questions to understand the WHY and HOW mechanisms like when the chronic process started, and how often the ulceration or inflammation increases and reduces. We measure data using the Subjective Unit of Distress 0-10 Scale which in unbelievably reliable in helping clients solidify what they feel, think or experience.[22]

Then we look at our Organ-Mind-Brain Anatomy™ Charts and read that the eczema is connected to the skin-epidermis tissue, that the psychosocial stress is mostly related to a loss-of-touch or separation type of conflictive life situations. The skin-epidermis symptoms change from pale, less sensitive skin symptoms in stress, to inflamed, itchy and hot symptoms during the regeneration process.

It's like each organ tissue symptom tells a personal story. If we really listed and know how to decode the symptom's message we can help our clients a lot faster and in a more profound way.

The Root-Cause Analysis main parameters for this eczema client (which was a real client of mine) read like this:

Symptom:	Eczema flaring up every 2-3 weeks
Organ Tissue:	Skin Epidermis
Stress:	Pale, numb, sensitive skin
Regeneration:	Inflamed, itchy, hot symptoms
Unresolved Emotion:	Fear (SUD 7)
Conflictive Thoughts:	Loss of child
Stress Trigger:	Divorce (fear of losing custody)

What's mind-blowing is that after this client realized the connection between her life situation and the eczema her skin-epidermis and psychosocial stress symptoms reduced by 50%.

---

[22] https://www.ncbi.nlm.nih.gov/pmc/articles/PMC4874244/

After two additional consultations over 4 weeks the eczema slowly reduced and disappeared completely.

Over these 4 weeks organ-tissue-specific Lifestyle Prescriptions® played an essential role.

One new psychosocial stress related habit agreed to be practice with the client was to be attentive and aware whenever the "separation-anxiety" type of emotions and thoughts get triggers. Practicing awareness and increasing the feelings of being in control and slowly (or fast) switching to a different habitual response made a huge difference for the client.

The Lifestyle Medicine approach would have absolutely worked too with the client practicing mindfulness, reducing overall stress and improving diet and social support. Change can happen in many ways.

But if we know that the specific "loss-of-touch" and "separation-anxiety" related to the looming divorce is directly linked to the skin-epidermis symptoms, helping this specific client was so much easier and quicker.

We saved time, costs and our clients typically look at us saying, *"How did you know what's going on in my mind and my life?"*

It's easy. Your body told me.

You might ask so what's the 3-Minute Lifestyle Prescriptions® Technique?

Dr. Kevin Chan, a very successful Family Medicine and Lifestyle Medicine practitioner with a super busy practice in Phoenix Arizona, is using Lifestyle Prescriptions® and Organ-Mind-Brain Anatomy™. Because he has only 5-15 minutes per client, he uses this protocol:

- A patient with eczema skin epidermis needs help

- He has two prescription pads ready.
- He asks the patient if they are open to address the Root-Cause of the eczema using evidence-based Lifestyle Medicine.
- Then he looks at the Organ-Mind-Brain Anatomy™ reference charts and shows the skin-epidermis chart to the patient saying, "Do you sometimes feel separation anxiety?"
- The patient looks at him with wide eyes saying, "How do you know?"
- Dr. Chan writes a Lifestyle Prescription® referral to a Health Coach in his office focused on reducing the psychosocial stress, unresolved emotions and conflictive thoughts as a first step to not just manage the symptom but addressing the root-cause and resolving the skin-epidermis organ tissue symptoms.

As you can see prescribing Lifestyle Medicine or organ-tissue-specific Lifestyle Prescriptions® is easy to do and your patients and clients will absolutely love you for it because they get better quickly.

Chapter Twelve

Johannes R. Fisslinger MA, LPHCS - Organ-Mind-Brain Anatomy™, the 6 Root-Causes and the Art and Science of Self-Healing

Johannes is the founder of Lifestyle Prescriptions® University, author of "The 6-Root-Causes of All Symptoms", and developer of the HealthiWealthi™ Coach Platform & Ecosystem. ↗ healthiwealthi.io

I want to share with you some of my work, and what I've been researching since the mind 1980s, which is most of my working life. But before that, I want to ask you something.

Go back a couple of days or weeks or months to when you had any chronic health condition.

If I would ask, how would you answer these questions?

- What was the specific symptom?
- Why did you get this symptom?
- What triggered or started it?
- Why did the symptom change, sometimes disappear and then return later with a vengeance?
- Which specific organ tissue was affected?
- Which symptoms have you noticed for that organ tissue during stress and in regeneration?
- Which specific stressful life situation, emotion, habitual conflictive thoughts were related to this chronic process?

The "WHY" is probably the most important question. You want to know what is going on and why this is happening to you. Why is it chronic? Why me? Why now?

There is a lot of information available these days about lifestyle medicine and the four pillars. I'd like to dive into this a bit deeper.

The four pillars of medicine are the primary approach in most non-conventional healthcare practices. They entail the consideration of sleep and stress management, physical activity, relationships, and nutrition. These are all areas to explore when asking the "why."

When I was about 18 or so, I had major conjunctivitis. It was really bad with my eyes continually burning like fire. This lasted for over two years, and then suddenly disappeared. During this time period, I kept asking myself, "Why is this happening to me? I'm only 18 and most young people don't usually suffer with such issues."

A few years later, I had major digestive issues. This led me to an interest in vegetarianism and healthy living habits, like yoga and mindfulness. Yet, my digestive issues continued for a while, eventually going away.

Twenty years later I suffered with some major, lower back pain. By this time, I was listening to my body better, being more conscious of pain before it got too bad and asking better questions. I understood the mind-body connections, and the importance of the "why" question. I knew by now that pain related to something going on in my life and wasn't just physical.

The mind-body connection showed me the mind had something going on and was manifesting in the body, the physical aspect of my being.

Once I made this mind-body connection, the pain went away within days and has never returned.

I began wondering, and even investigating, if there is a model available to help individuals better understand the mind-body connection, and the art and science of self-healing. I knew this was needed for root-cause analysis purposes to better help individuals, as well as professionals, with proper diagnostics.

If you look at human biology, you can see it is something more complicated than our conscious mind can easily comprehend. As you know, we all have a fight-or-flight response to our own individual triggers. Once we are aware of these triggers, we can start becoming mindful of the symptoms. We then grow in our understanding working towards auto-regulation and healing.

The point is there are these six root causes that have a powerful effect on our health and our life. Once we start to realize what these root causes are, and we can feel it in our body, we can connect with it. We realize we can increase awareness and recognize what these specific root-causes are.

We start noticing that something triggered us into stress with specific emotions and thoughts swirling around inside of us. We might feel very sad with habitual-automated thoughts and memories about a looming separation.

We might feel upset and constantly think about the fight with our boss that wants to tell me what to do (which is difficult to digest). At the same time, we also feel our heart rate increase, sweaty palms, and other stress related symptoms plus to our surprise our stomach is really tight, highly pain and a feeling of sensitive. We start realizing that something needs to be done now to prevent this to develop further into a full-blown crisis.

Over the last twenty years, research has been making process in understanding the mind-body, the brain-gut, and the gut-microbiome connection.[23]

Our work and teachings at Lifestyle Prescriptions® are deeply rooted in Organ-Mind-Brain Anatomy™ and the empirically verified knowledge that specific stressors, emotions, and thoughts/beliefs and lifestyle habits are directly linked and impact specific organ tissues with different type of symptoms showing in the stress and regeneration phase.

Let's unpack this statement.

THE 6 ROOT-CAUSES

Once we look at ourselves as a complex organism that constantly reacts, interacts and responds to internal and external stimuli and information then we'll start seeing a variety of root-cause(s).

All of us tend to look for "the one root-cause" or reason that is triggers or causes symptoms. But the reality is there are six possible root-causes that we need to address.

These 6 Root-Cause(s) are:

1. Organ
2. Stress
3. Emotion
4. Belief
5. Social
6. Lifestyle

---

[23] https://www.lifestyleprescriptions.tv/phd/research-science/

Here's how you can think about the 6 Root-Cause(s) using a Smartphone metaphor:

1. **ORGAN**: Physical smartphone with all its components, parts, subparts and wiring.
2. **STRESS**: What or who is causing the malfunction? What puts stress on the specific phone components? What is the trigger?
3. **EMOTION**: It's the intensity and repetition of the electricity or energy that is running through the device. The more repetition and the higher the charge, the stronger symptoms will show up.
4. **BELIEF**: The operating system that works behind the scene and regulates 90% of the phone's processes.
5. **SOCIAL**: People that use, interact and are influenced by the smartphone.
6. **LIFESTYLE**: How well do we take care of the device? Do we maintain the hardware and upgrade the software regularly? Do we protect it from damage? [24]

Think about you as a synchronous organism where you with these 6 sublevels are directly linked with your life. Our software (emotions, thoughts, perceptions) is directly links via our brain and nervous system with our organs (tissues) which in turn feedback to our brain and our mind. [25]

The beauty though is that this process is not random at all but highly intelligent and biological meaningful which means all

---

[24] Excerpt from the book The 6 Root-Causes of all Symptoms, Johannes R. Fisslinger

[25] https://www.lifestyleprescriptions.tv/phd/research-science/

symptoms we experience are part of an innate survival and auto-regulation mechanism that is meant to help us deal with life

How brilliant is this. We suddenly can relax a bit (which does not mean doing nothing…) and perceive the beauty of our bodily vehicle as something to be proud of (followed by conscious actions to get return the organ tissues showing symptoms back into balance.).

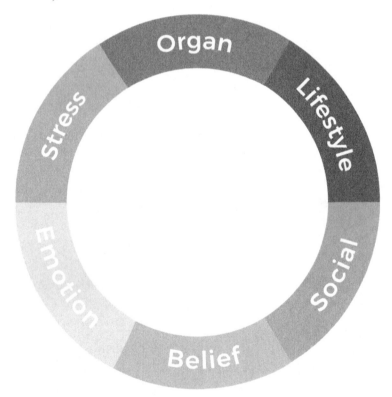

Being clear about which organ tissue is reacting and showing symptoms is important because it tells us about the biological function of that organ tissue. It also shows us what we're feeling

and thinking and which type of biological conflict we have experienced.

The thin skin-epidermis layer has biologically and physiologically completely different purpose and function compared to the thick skin-dermis layer.

The eyes are very complex with over 10 unique "parts" or organ tissues including the retina, vitreous body, cornea, iris, macula, lens, sclera, conjunctiva and others. Every one of these eye organ tissues has a different purpose and function in our body which in turn means the type of stress affecting them is uniquely different.

We could just look at the organ (skin, liver, lungs or eyes), but being more specific and defining which organ tissue is affected is going to take us a huge step further.

- SKIN: Is it the epidermis, dermis or subcutaneous tissue?
- LIVER: Parenchyma, or gall bladder gland or ducts?
- LUNGS: Bronchial mucosa, goblet cells or alveoli?
- EYES: Retina, vitreous body, cornea or crystalline lens?

Use these foundational questions to explore the deeper meaning of organ tissue symptoms:

- What's the biological function of this organ tissue?
- What's the physiological or anatomical function?
- Why did this specific tissue react?
- What type of life situation or biological theme could be involved?

THE MAJOR POINTS & PHASES OF SELF-HEALING

If self-healing sounds to unscientific, then please use the terms auto-regulation or homeostasis. We're talking about a natural, inherent process that allows our body, and each specific organ tissue, to return to its natural state.

One of the most effective tools we use in our Lifestyle Prescriptions® Root-Cause Analysis Process related to the HOW and the TIMELINE which means how each organ tissue processes from the start to the end of a chronic process.

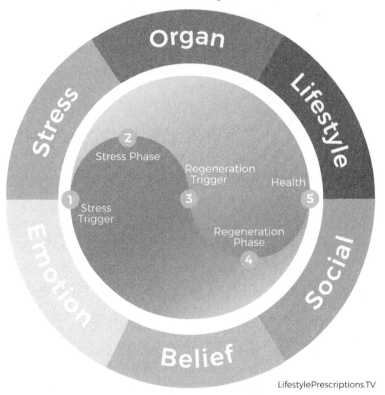

Again, this process is not random either. It's pretty specific. The simplified, main points and phases of this organ tissue auto-regulation process are:

1. **STRESS TRIGGER**
   - Unexpected, highly emotional, often traumatic life situations that trigger a fight-flight-freeze response
   - Or small sensory habitual trigger (something we see,

hear, smell, taste, feel or think) retriggering old memories and habitual Organ-Mind-Brain reactions)

2. **STRESS**   **PHASE**
   - Increased sympathetic activity, hormone levels, high emotions, conflictive thoughts and organ-tissue-specific symptoms (like pale, white, flaky epidermis skin)

3. **REGENERATION**   **TRIGGER**
   - There are several ways how Organ-Mind-Brain may switch from sympathetic to parasympathetic activity as part of the repair and regeneration process.
   - Typically, the conflictive situation has resolved, we decided to let go of it, we had a good night rest, or the trigger is not present anymore.

4. **REGENERATION**   **PHASE**
   - Increased parasympathetic activity with a variety of symptoms like feeling sick, hot, fever, fatigue, exhaustion, need to sleep, brain fog, increased microbial activity with organ-tissue-specific repair symptoms (like red, hot inflamed and itchy epidermis skin).

5. **HEALTH**
   - Our organism has returned to homeostasis, the auto-regulation process is complete (depending on other factors including lifestyle either with a full or partial recovery).

The big challenge with Chronic Symptoms is the retrigger process because typically we repeat the same 5-step chronic cycle again and again.

Monday, we go back to the hated work place and are triggered by just seeing our hated co-worker (8+ hours stress phase). When we leave work daily and have a good night sleep we somewhat regenerate and wake up with a headache (regeneration phase symptom).

Not knowing Organ-Mind-Brain Anatomy™ we don't realize that the exhaustion, fatigue, feel sick with fever and migraine that hit us Friday evening is part of that deeper regeneration that our organism needs to recover from the high-stress work days.

Another example is a mother blaming herself for her 7-year young child bedwetting every time she returned from the divorced fathers weekend stay. She believed it was her fault because the child never peed into her bed while staying with her dad. After a quick root-cause analysis it was clear that the child did not want to go to the dad, felt tremendous internal pressure and not "at home", like she does in her mom's house own room.

Bedwetting is related typically to the bladder mucosa which from a biological perspective relates to our personal space, our territory or identity that we want to but can't define.

Hence, the bedwetting in the regeneration phase when the stressful situation was over and she was safely back at home.

This is just one of many examples why knowing the timeline of chronic symptoms is essential in a targeted and root-cause-based Lifestyle Medicine and Health Coaching Practice.

Becoming an expert and specialist in eliciting the 6 Root-Causes and Points & Phases of Self-Healing and using evidence-based Lifestyle Medicine and Health Coaching protocols will be foundational tools for all healthcare practitioners in the future.

Why?

Because Lifestyle Medicine works. And it works a lot better, knowing and mastering Organ-Mind-Brain Anatomy™.

Chapter Thirteen

Aisling Killoran - Psychosocial Stressors and Infertility (New Research)

Aisling Killoran is a Root-Cause Health Coach Specialist™, Lifestyle Prescriptions® University Faculty Member with over 20 years' experience in health and wellness, focusing on psychosocial support strategies for unexplained infertility. ⭧ accomplishchange.net

Let us start this discussion with a story. This story tells about the journey of Mary, a pseudonym that represents the journey of many women who have been trying to conceive.

Mary had two wishes. The first was to meet her life partner, which she did at age 38. And the second was to have a baby. Like many women, Mary was trying to conceive for over two years when she reached out for help. Her medical assessments came back clear, with a prognosis of unexplained infertility.

Mary had three avenues to explore.

1) Continuing her path of evaluating her lifestyle, nutrition, diet, and exercise programs.

2) Investigating in-vitro fertilization (IVF). (She decided to give herself three to six months before she would embark on this option.)

3) Explore more deeply her lifestyle, diet, exercise, and sleep, as well as the emotional aspects of her life.

What did Mary decide? Her burning desire to have a baby was so strong that she decided to look at the emotional areas that were yet unexplored. This could offer clues to any obstacles preventing her from conceiving. During her exploration Mary uncovered some subconscious blocks that she chose to address. These psychosocial stressors were a combination of negative emotions, personal conflicts, limiting beliefs, and self-sabotaging behaviors.

Mary had two very strong negative emotions. One was sadness, which is understandable as she had been trying to conceive for quite some time. And the second was grief. The deepening grief of not getting pregnant as each month passed by. Mary was "feeling into" the experience of a lot of grief in her life from not being able to conceive, rather than tuning into the joy of motherhood.

In addition to the negative emotions, Mary also experienced two very strong life complications. One was loss. Mary experienced a lot of loss during her life. As a child, she lost some siblings. As a teenager, she lost one parent after losing the other years earlier. So, there was a lot of loss in Mary's life, along with the loss of dreams. Mary also decided to put her career on hold while trying to conceive which brought about the loss of future career opportunities.

Mary also experienced physical and sexual abuse as an adolescent. In addition to the negative emotions and life complexities, Mary had some very strong limiting beliefs. Her first belief was, "I've waited too long." The second belief was, "It's my fault." The third belief was, "I feel like a failure." Mary had these three very strong limiting beliefs. Again, she also had some self-sabotaging programs that she had gotten really good at running in the background of her thoughts. The saboteurs were, "I don't deserve to be pregnant." "It's not safe for me to be pregnant." And, "I'm not worthy of being pregnant." These were very strong beliefs that Mary held deep, all needing released.

Working with Mary as her health coach, we explored her emotional issues. We used solution-focused intervention techniques that fall under the umbrella of energy psychology.

Together, we addressed her emotional landscape using an Emotional Freedom Technique known as Emotional Freedom Tapping (EFT). This method was used to manage her beliefs around her inability to conceive.

As we progressed, we used hypnosis and guided visualization to help Mary connect with her womb and reproductive system to improve and enhance this relationship. This was because Mary's relationship with her reproductive parts was one, she never connected well with. Hence, we used guided visualization to enhance her connection with her womb. We worked through this journey together, through nine months of pregnancy, and into a great birthing experience.

In addition to hypnosis, the Tapas Acupressure Technique (TAT) was also incorporated into her healing. This method addressed the traumas of Mary's life, predominantly the losses, along with the physical and sexual abuses that she experienced as an adolescent. In addition to this technique was cognitive reframing where we took Mary's core sabotaging beliefs and reframed them. This switched her beliefs into knowing that she deserved to have a baby, that she was worthy of having a baby, and that it was her time to have a baby.

We continued with Lifestyle Prescriptions® and health coaching. Mary was coached on connecting to her body and addressing all the stresses she was experiencing from her past beliefs, lifestyle, and social interactions. All these interventions that were incorporated throughout her healing journey are part of Lifestyle Prescriptions® protocol.

As a result of working through this process with not just Mary but eight other women, we had a 72% success rate. We know that Mary is not alone in her struggle to conceive. There are thousands of women who experience high mental and emotional stress levels that contribute to "unexplained" infertility. How can we bridge this gap in helping others like Mary achieve their dreams?

The demographics of our six-month study was women between the ages of 34-40 with a focus on these areas:

- Limiting beliefs- False beliefs as a result of incorrect assumptions
- Conflicts in belief systems- Not having a full grasp on one's own personal beliefs
- Stressors- A perceived challenging event

What did we discover about emotions, conflicts, beliefs, and sabotage with our research group? The strongest negative emotions were:

- Pain
- Anger
- Sadness
- Grief
- Shame
- Hurt
- Fear
- Frustration

It is easy to understand where the emotional and physical pain comes from with women desiring to conceive.

Physical pain is many times a result of emotional discomfort. Physical pain can be anything from tightness in the chest to a tight knot in the stomach. We can see why these ladies experienced considerable emotional pain around not being able to conceive.

In addition to pain, there was a tremendous amount of anger. They were angry at themselves. They were angry at those around them who were pregnant. And they were also angry just at life in general because they were not getting pregnant. Adding to the anger was a considerable amount of shame. They felt shame within themselves for not being able to conceive. They were out with their friends who had children while they didn't have any children. They had other pregnant family members, and they felt so ashamed that they were not pregnant as well. They thought they were letting their families down, which made them feel a huge amount of shame.

Then there was sadness- the sadness of not being pregnant and the possible loss of a journey of not having children. Also, there was grief around not being pregnant yet, along with the grief of loss around missing out on having children. Another emotion was fear, and a considerable amount was present. The fear was from not getting pregnant to what would be involved with getting pregnant. Also, there was the fear of going through nine months of pregnancy and the possibility of miscarriage. So, there was a vast amount of fear and frustration in addition to the many other emotional upsets. These nine ladies had experienced a lot of frustration, which is quite understandable.

Adding to the eight negative emotions were other very strong life conflicts. The first of these five was the decreased quality of life. These ladies withdraw from life in general by reducing their contacts with friends, family, and colleagues. They withdraw from social interaction from family and friends because they felt embarrassed that they didn't have children. They also felt ashamed and jealous because they would see their friends pregnant when they were out with them. So, they made decisions to pull back even more on visiting their friends and family as time went on. They turned down social events and even christenings due to the upset, the shame, and the fear that they felt.

Another challenge they had was a huge amount of loss from:

- Not being pregnant.

- Not fulfilling their dreams.
- Opportunity loss with not having children at a younger age.
- Time away from their career as they took a break to concentrate on conceiving.

Then there was more fear around their pregnancy and self-devaluation. Self-devaluation is very important to recognize because these ladies were beating themselves up, feeling that they were not good enough, or that their bodies had failed them. They felt a considerable amount of internal pressure, and did a lot of negative thinking about themselves.

We also discover that, across the board, each study participant had some degree of physical and/or sexual abuse in their history. With some, it was childhood experiences and with others it involved relationships with past partners.

Adding to the sexual and physical abuse was sexual conflict. The sexual conflict resulted from past toxic relationships that got them very stressed around issues of conceiving. The fact that the windows were closing as the years were going by, and with each passing month finding themselves not pregnant, was putting a huge amount of pressure on the couples. From a sexual relation perspective, a lot of stress and conflict from the past presented itself, with some of the ladies having vulvodynia (unexplained vaginal pain), or vaginitis (inflammation and pain in the vaginal area).

Questioning them further showed some powerful limiting beliefs. There were 32 limiting beliefs, with five core ones:

- It is my fault I cannot get pregnant.
- I am too busy to get pregnant.
- I have waited too long for the opportunity.
- It is not safe for me to get pregnant.

- I feel like a failure.

They also had strong self-sabotaging tendencies as Mary did, including:

- I don't deserve to be pregnant.
- I am not worthy of getting pregnant.
- I don't trust my body to get pregnant.
- It is not safe for me to get pregnant.

These are all intense emotions, conflicts, limiting beliefs, and self-sabotaging tendencies these ladies had in common.

Our research made it clear that women who experience unexplained infertility presented high levels of mental and emotional stress that contributes to their inability to conceive.

Most medical doctors cannot pinpoint 23% of circumstances around unexplained infertility resulting from psychosocial stressors as an underlying factor. They don't address unexplained infertility issues like limiting beliefs, lifestyle choices, emotional upsets, or negative thinking.

My colleagues and I at Lifestyle Prescriptions® University have spent years looking deeply into these aspects behind unexplained infertility.

We are now at a point to asking a big question. How do we most optimally balance psychosocial stress using the four pillars of Lifestyle Medicine?

Our assessments with many clients show that a lot of them look only at areas of nutrition and exercise. The best approach is looking at a balanced combination of all aspects of health. We need to look at what someone is currently doing, and what areas are being neglected. Next, we look at the emotional issues of each individual since this is the area least wanting to be addressed. How can we incorporate this into lifestyle changes?

Sometimes women exercise but hate they type of exercising they are doing. This would cause more stress and negative feelings then any positive results. Asking individuals what exercise they really enjoy doing is important. They might simply say, "Well, I prefer just walking." We can then suggest, "Why don't you change the exercise you're doing from running at the gym to walking instead?"

Sometimes it can be the little, simple changes that make a huge difference. This goes for nutrition as well as exercise. It could be a simple thing like reducing the intake of coffee because caffeine, or rather too much caffeine, isn't healthy when you are trying to conceive.

Many women come to me, and as part of my examining procedure, I always ask if they have been down the medical route. I want to be sure to have a medical assessment ensuring that the infertility reason is coming back diagnosed as unexplained. As mentioned earlier, 23% of people who come to see us have no circumstances that could be identified as contributing to their infertility. This is where my work begins with the women in these circumstances.

There are a lot of connections between emotions, stress, beliefs, lifestyle, and habits. From a lifestyle and social perspective, another aspect of our group of women we noted was their blocking themselves off from society; they pulled back, they didn't go out much anymore, and the joy from social support seemed to diminish.

One of the most important things that I encourage my clients to do is to start meeting their friends for a walk, a catch-up, lunch, or even just a phone call for a quick conversation. I might even give them a lifestyle prescription to go on date nights with their partner.

The emphasis with the clients is that they need to conjure up joy back into their lives. They need to go on dates with their partners and start having fun again. Even from a sexual relations perspective, all the fun can be gone from that. It is all about encouraging them to get back in action and have fun and do the things they used to do before they started focusing on conceiving.

The practical applications that I work with clients, specifically lifestyle medicine and health coaching, addresses lifestyle factors of diet, nutrition, exercise, and stress management. Lifestyle Prescriptions® incorporates tools in getting women to imagine that they can get pregnant.

We also want to incorporate some cognitive reframing when we hear remarks like, "Every time I read social media, I see people who are pregnant, and I am so jealous." They don't like feeling jealous, yet they are. In this case we would ask them to "reframe" with phrases like, "I'll be pregnant next!" Simple phrases like this are very affirming.

We can also adopt specific, simple, lifestyle modifications. Like I said before, every time they are out and about, and they see somebody else pregnant, they should say, "I'm next." That's one effortless thing they can do. Another helpful exercise for them is to visualize themselves being pregnant. Some people say they can't do that, and this would require finding another method that works for them.

At times I've encouraged clients to go and buy a pair of baby socks or a small item of clothing. This is something so simple, yet effective to the psyche. I've had women come back to me and tell me they did this, and how it lifted their mood. The objective of this simple, little exercise is to have them believe that they have a little baby fitting into those socks. Sometimes, I will ask these anxious women to look in the mirror and talk to themselves, saying things like, "You know what, I've got this, our baby is on its way. We can do this!"

Another helpful practice is to get them to communicate with their partners and have conversations about sexual relations. They need to do this, to get out there and reignite their sexual relationship. A lot of the time it's non-existent outside of ovulation, and this is sad.

Another thing that's important yet so very simple, is having date nights. With the women in our studies focusing only on conceiving, a big portion of their lives went on hold. Getting out and having fun can be healing. This is the most important prescription we can write them. It's vital to get back out there and have fun.

This also applies to those with other health issues along with the unexplained infertility. You'll be working with people who have a medical diagnosis around why they're not conceiving, and the only route for them is IVF. The stress that they go through can be catastrophic.

Ideally, there is help for these women, but they don't always realize it. And mostly they tend to not think about any emotional components. They don't do this intentionally. They just don't think about it and it's not something others think of or will want to discuss. I believe huge stress levels go along the IVF route. And these women, for whatever reason, did not stop to think that if they addressed the emotional components, it could make significant improvements to their fertility journey with or without IVF. Along with nutrition, exercise, diet, and social support, emotional issues and stress need addressed. This is important because when we fail to address the psychosocial stress, emotions, beliefs, thoughts, and values, we miss key components along the healing journey.

Another issue I've been mentioned is isolation. Intentionally or unintentionally, these women put themselves into isolation. The opposite of this is actually the most supportive - come out of isolation, meet with friends and family, attend gatherings, even small ones.

It's the quantum steps that make a difference.

You harness small habits, small positive changes, and that's what's important to conquering any health issue.

Chapter Fourteen

Annie Gedye B.Sc., LPHCS - The 9 Points and Phases of *Chronic Symptoms and the Autonomic Nervous System*

Annie Gedye is a Root-Cause Health Coach Specialist™ (LPHCS) and Lifestyle Prescriptions® University Faculty Member with over 33 years in the health and wellness industry.

Let's look at the nine points and phases of chronic symptoms and how the autonomic nervous system is involved. This is central, and one of my most favorite things about the autonomic nervous system.

What if... what you think health and illness are all about, especially what causes chronic illness, was something totally different? We know that about 80% of all health problems in the world today are chronic issues. Chronic diseases are non-communicable issues like arthritis, eczema, type 2 diabetes, heart disease, cancer, and multiple sclerosis. We also know that prolonged stress can make us ill. Most people are familiar with this information since it is scientific, specific, and can be applied to the general population.

We all have access to the same health information and advice. But there is a way to make the information very personal and specific to you and your clients, and this is what we will explore.

To understand the cause of chronic illness, we need an introduction to the autonomic nervous system before we look at the nine points and phases that help us track the symptoms. We need to know what the autonomic nervous system is doing. Then we can link it to chronic symptoms. We can define the autonomic nervous system as, "The part of the nervous system responsible for the control of the bodily functions not consciously directed-breathing, heartbeat, and digestive processes."

We experience life as a rhythm between polarities.

The first step to exploring the nine points and phases of self-healing is understanding how sickness and chronic disease manifests, and to accept that these natural opposites and fluctuations occur. The autonomic nervous system is classically divided into two systems- the parasympathetic and the sympathetic. Each operates independently in some functions, and in cooperation with others. Sometimes the enteric nervous system is included; referred to as the second brain.

Our body's autonomic nervous system has a quick response that mobilizes our fight, flight, or freeze response. The parasympathetic is more slowly activated and offers a dampening system in many cases, to counter the fight-flight-freeze. One will activate a physiological response and the other one inhibits it. In our work, we call the sympathetic nervous system, "the stress phase," and parasympathetic, "the regeneration phase." There is a natural flow from one to the other. One does not operate without the other.

How and why does this autonomic nervous system cycle work, and how does it heal and cause chronic illness? How is that even possible? In 1997, Dr. Candace Pert wrote and published an iconic book *Molecules of Emotion: The Science Behind Mind-Body Medicine.* She is often referred to as the mother of psychoneurosis immunology. In essence, her groundbreaking work shows that our cell surfaces are aligned with many specific receptors to which only specific molecules can attach themselves. More specifically her extensive work in the field explains how specific molecules, the neuropeptides, carry emotional messages throughout the body and can change the chemistry of every cell.

You can think about it this way, good emotions enhance our activity, and negative emotions are damaging.

One quote in her book states, "When emotions are expressed... all systems are united and made whole. When emotions are repressed, denied, not allowed to be whatever they may be, our network pathways get blocked, stopping the flow of the vital feel-good, unifying chemicals that run both our biology and our behavior."

Her work made it clear how emotions can be key to understanding disease. This is very important because it is crucial in our understanding of all illnesses, most importantly, chronic diseases. Many processes controlled by the autonomic nervous system are unconscious or involuntary, like breathing, heart rate, salivation, and digestion. How can knowing about the autonomic nervous system help us understand illnesses and chronic diseases?

Imagine this cycle:

---

1. A stress response comes from an emotional trigger.
2. This invokes chemical responses within us, like adrenaline and cortisol.

If the cycle continues looping through 1 stress phase and 2 regeneration phases, our physiology will eventually respond with chronic illness.

1, 2, 1, 2, 1, 2, 1, 2, 1, 2 = Chronic Illness

At the sympathetic system, we have the response which mobilizes our body to react to real or perceived danger and initiate the fight, flight, or freeze mechanisms. These are survival mechanisms. And in our natural rhythm of polarities, in the daytime, this is when we have the sympathetic response, with its active period from 6:00 a.m. until 8 p.m. Natural rhythm means-active, being awake, and functioning normally. This provides enough energy to do our daily tasks. This is not the phenetic hair-on-end, high stress, that we all experience from time to time.

Some typical sympathetic responses that we observe in this state when we are in high stress from an event, or just when we have a little bit of a fretful time, or when we've got a conditioned reflex and the conditioned reflex is something that we just keep responding to in the same way.

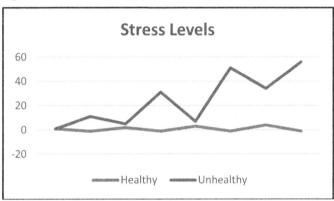

When we are experiencing a stress state, (as shown in chart above) we are stressed in our physical body- maybe with sore shoulders, aching muscles, obsessive thinking, and the monkey mind.

We could experience any of these symptoms:

- Sleeplessness
- Loss of appetite
- Fluctuation of body temperature
- Cold or hot extremities
- High blood pressure
- Shallow breathing
- Cold sweats

Any of these symptoms could happen in response to a real or perceived threat of trauma and gear us up to survival through our biology.

Let's take a look at what's involved with these two different systems.

PARASYMPATHETIC	SYMPATHETIC
Activated slowly	Quick responder
Allows for repair and cellular regeneration	Fatigue and tiredness
Natural recovery happens at night between 8 p.m. and 6 a.m.	Hunger and weight gain
Regeneration- Sleeping and recuperating	Warm body, inflammation, low blood pressure, slow heart rate. When extreme- fever and severe inflammation become chronic
Buildup of resources	Mentally fuzzy
Digestive organs active- stomach, bowel, liver	Microbes and viruses very active

Hans Selye, a Hungarian endocrinologist, developed the stress model called the "general adaptation syndrome." This concept thoroughly explains the stress response and how aging and disease are caused by chronic stress exposure. He noticed that the body adapts to external stresses in a predictable, biological pattern so internal balance is restored and maintained, which results in an overall healthy system.

Any stress response should only be very short-lived. Think animals. A deer is chased by a lion but gets away. What does it do? It shakes itself off and continues on. The stress is gone. It happens that quick. We humans however tend to hang on to and continue repeating the process with memory triggers. Chronic illness doesn't come from an isolated stressful incident but chronic, prolonged, or regular exposure to the triggers causing a repeated stress response in the body. It's like our worst version of the movie Groundhog Day. These triggers are through our senses-seeing, hearing, touching, smelling, or tasting, and leading to negative self-talk. You know that monkey mind when you just can't let go of something. It's not only about the actual stressor or life event that has happened. Very importantly, it's about our perception of it, and how we respond emotionally to it. This affects our response if it's a real stressor or not.

Remember Dr. Pert's scientific observations about the connection of emotions and disease? Hans Selye also noticed that if a stress is not resolved, there is a very chronic stress state that develops where we remain on high alert. And we adapt and live with higher stress levels. This is typical of so many in society today. It results in our bodies going through changes that we are unaware of in an attempt to cope with stress.

We continue to secrete stress hormones and our blood pressure can remain high. We may think that we are managing our stress well, but our body's physical responses show a different scenario. If the stress stage goes on too long without resolution, then we go into the exhaustion stage and with such low vitality that our body does not have the resources to heal itself. At that very low ebb, we may feel hopeless and want to give up. We may be so fatigued that we can hardly move. At this stage, we feel burned-out, depressed, anxious, and less tolerance of nearly everything. Most importantly, our immune system weakens, and we become at risk to any number of stress-related illnesses that we see manifesting all around us. This is where lifestyle interventions, such as nutrition, are so very important to help the body increase vitality and produce the energy to support healing.

Our health story is dynamic. It is a dynamic state of adaptation to life when we move into a stress trigger. This is the cause of our chronic and acute symptoms, and we'll learn more about this as we step through the process. Remember, the stress-trigger can be a real or a perceived trauma, event, or a conditioned response. When responding to an unexpected traumatic event, we usually have no conscious strategy in place to deal with it. Our unconscious survival mechanism takes over with a solution or strategy to ensure survival. This is when we go into the stress phase, which is the fight, flight, or freeze response. It's an unconscious, predictable, biological pattern.

We also notice the symptoms evident in the sympathetic phase that we talked about earlier. The internal conflicts causing over-thinking, feeling cold, not sleeping well, blood pressure fluctuations, and obsessive emotional takeover. This all causes increased stress hormones which can lead to illness, either in this phase, or more often in the regeneration phase. Physical illnesses in the stress phase could be something like high blood pressure that a person already experiences, only to an increased degree. It's naturally there with a constant release of stress hormones. Some people experience stomach ulcers. Be aware that not all stress-induced illnesses occur in the stress phase.

Interestingly, most illnesses show up in the next phase, the regeneration phase. This follows the stress phase like day follows night. This is a predictable, biological pattern. The stress phase is an essential forerunner and cause of the manifestation of the regeneration symptoms which we call the illness. Stress is at the bottom of all our symptoms in one way or another, manifesting directly or indirectly in the regeneration phase.

Moving from the stress stage to the regeneration phase actually moves toward symptoms of "unhealth." This is how the autonomic nervous system allows healing to occur. How and why does this happen? It's the body's natural way to transition into healing. Regeneration trigger can be a real-life solution. We could leave a difficult job, complete a complicated college program, or have an inner transformation. A total internal shift could leads to a permanent behavioral response. Any particular stress trigger can bring about a change. With an understanding of this transition, we can learn to avoid such traumatic experiences in the future.

Another issue about chronic illness is the matter of conflicts being "passive." Unfortunately, this is very common. This means that the trauma response can be triggered at any time, day, week, month, or even years after an initial trauma. There is usually a temporary resolution but not a solution. Maybe, just sleeping on it makes you feel better or maybe you are in denial, or that stressor is just not present in your life at the moment. Sometimes you can say, "I don't have the time to deal with it now" and then suppress it. That is not healthy. So, passive conflicts resolution explains why we are triggered chronically and have chronic illness symptoms.

You can see how easy it is to tell which state you're in. This is something we can all do. Stress phase or regeneration phase. It just takes a little observation to feel what is happening in your body. If you find yourself with monkey mind, ask yourself what just happened? The stressor could be something that is only momentarily, like a stressful phone call. Maybe you have to cancel an event that someone else was looking forward to? But after you do it, how do you feel? You take a sigh of relief, and a deep breath. That's the opposite of the shallow breathing which occurs in the stress phase. All day long we are moving from the stress to the regeneration phase. It's the flow of life. How often have we worked our socks off in the sympathetic stress phase to get away for our two-week holiday, only to get flu the first day of our vacation?

More about the parasympathetic regeneration symptoms. The first part is when people seek help to get relief from symptoms. With conventional medicine, in the regeneration symptom phase, symptoms of an illness are often acute but can turn chronic. We know that medications are only used to treat symptoms and not the root-cause of the physical distress.

With the damage done to our physiology in the stress phase, symptoms worsen. If high stress dissipates, hormone levels repair. As the body is repairing, we feel sick with fatigue, inflammation, increased metabolism, and more microbial and viral activity throughout the body. Manifestations of these symptoms could be a cold, flu, arthritis, back or shoulder pain, eczema, all with inflammation. These parasympathetic symptoms usually include mind-fog as it forces people into a resting stage to enable repair.

Usually, we think of sickness and symptoms as one. We think we are either on or off, well or sick. This is not so. With using the nine points and phases, we differentiate these symptoms into different phases of the autonomic nervous system. A stressful regeneration phase will follow a stressful stress phase; there is direct relationship degree between the stress and the recovery. Small stressors have a shorter, less traumatic recovery, whereas a severe childhood trauma could take years to recover from, emotionally as well as physically.

Reeducating students and clients present big challenges. Understanding that the root cause of illness is a stress trigger event that activates natural, predictable, biological patterns and cycles is a different way of thinking about health and wellness.

200

"Reframing" is one method we teach at Lifestyle Prescriptions® University to help shift the understanding in health beliefs and interpreting symptoms.

It is an "AHA" moment to our realization that what we thought all of our lives might be incorrect. With this understanding we see that symptoms are not isolated, random occurrences coming out of nowhere. It's part of a biologically, meaningful process with a start, middle, and end.

Our nine-phase system helps empower people to realize there is hope in resolving chronic as well as acute health issues. This can only happen with a true willingness for change.

The healing peak is a very short sympathetic stress phase. It can be seconds or hours, depending on the organ tissues involved, and it mostly goes unnoticed.

After the first six phases the body moves into the Regeneration B Phase. In this phase the body starts to normalize. At this point a person has a sense that they have turned the corner with their illness and that their body is moving towards regained health. The organ functions start to normalize but due to the internal scarring there is excretions of waste from repairing cells. The waste is dispensed mostly through urination, so this is a symptom to be aware of.

The amount of scarring of the internal organs will depend on the intensity and length of the stress regeneration cycles. With chronic situations, organ tissue function could be compromised making it less flexible and harder to recover. To support cell repair and vitality, it is important to eat live, whole foods, and engage in some gentle exercise, preferably outside. Any other self-care that a person can do will help quicken the recovery.

Moving through the phases, phase eight is the point where a person feels well again. This is when the system has normalized.

And in phase nine, we're back into the natural auto-regulatory flow and the rhythm of life's little ups and downs. This is how the autonomic cycle maintains our health.

Through the nine points and phases, we can find, and then with therapy modalities, resolve the destructive emotions and beliefs from the root cause of the trauma event, which triggers the stress phase. We can then break the cycle of this constant triggering which creates chronic symptoms. The body can heal itself naturally by normalizing and self-regulating. The symptoms very often resolve or greatly diminish depending on how long they've been in the retrigger cycle. If it was decades, it will take a longer time. This is how chronic events happen, as I've mentioned earlier.

1) Real or perceived threat or trauma, even a memory of one.
2) Emotional retrigger, a conditional reflex, like Pavlov's dog. The trigger can be a place, a voice tone, certain lighting, a food, a smell, or anything involved to stimulate the negative emotions which starts the stress response.
Each time these patterns repeat, the symptoms worsen.

In summary, as health coaches, we aim to help release the stress trigger responses and the emotions that go with it. This stops the stress and physiological response in the body from the original event replaying over and over again. This frees the client from the chronic cycle and helps prepare the body to heal.

I understand as a lifestyle medicine practitioner the high importance of the basic cornerstones - nutrition, movement, sleep, love and support, and stress management. If we apply these fundamentals, as well as work with and release stress trigger responses, we can help increase vitality and allow the body to heal. This is a well-rounded approach to lifestyle medicine.

We are not victims of disease.

Our symptoms are rather a biologically meaningful processes that are miraculously protecting us as part of our survival mechanism. As we and our clients become aware of the natural rhythm, a lot of fear about illnesses is also released. With this understanding we can find ways to balance our bodies, increase our vitality, and help our bodies to self-regulate and self-heal naturally.

Chapter Fifteen

Yasmine Farouk MA, LPHCS - The Emotion-Body Roller Coaster

Yasmine Farouk is one of the leading teachers of mental health, family development, and psychology across the Middle East and Europe. She is a Psycho-Spiritual Fitness Coach and Neuroplasticity Instructor, founder of ALTC in the Middle East, a faculty member at Lifestyle Prescriptions® University, and is currently working on her MS in Clinical Psychology.

This discussion on the "emotion-body roller coaster" is basically to explain what happens when we feel certain kinds of emotions, and what transpires internally as a response. As we know, there is a link between emotions and logic, including psychosomatic experiences.

The body is continuously urged to seek what is called comatose - a state where the body does not need to do any extra effort. Of course, too comatose would be a flat line, or dead. But keeping close to an even baseline is ideal. Here, the body is always trying to keep everything on autopilot, not wanting any intruders, and everything running smoothly. Not wanting anything that would make the body use excess energy.

Homeostasis, in biology, refers to optimal functioning.

It is a state of continued balance that happens internally, physically, and chemically, to keep the body on an even keel. If a body goes into a high or low swing, we know it will reverse, always attempting to keep at a steady baseline. Our body does not work alone though; the body and the psyche work together. Our body listens to what's going on in our minds. It is always searching for new kinds of signals from our emotional being. These signals are called our emotional print.

If we could graph emotional prints as healthy or unhealthy, we would come up with something like this. We can see two distinct cycles.

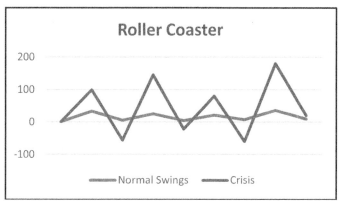

We can ask ourselves at any time, "What is my emotional print?" The question basically is to help us recognize how we are feeling, or what is our emotional state at this very moment? Are we feeling…?

- Excited
- Happy
- Scared
- Sad
- Angry

The body is very sensitive to emotional signals, and this creates our ever-changing emotional print.

This emotional print sets off signals, and the body respects and responds to these signals. For example, I eat all the right foods to be healthy. But if my body listens to signals of sadness, anger, or fear, my balance or homeostasis will be out of alignment with good health. If my emotional signals are feelings of happiness, joy, or excitement, my body will be in a state of balanced homeostasis and health. In this case, the body says, "All good.

Check, check. Keep going. Everything is fine. No problems!" We feel good in this state, we feel energized, we are active, and our mind is clear. We make good decisions, we provide solid support to others, and we feel good about life.

It is easy to solve problems when there is harmony between the mind, soul, and body. But what if the opposite happens? What if the not-so-good emotions set in and cause a mind-body disconnect? Of course, this is normal at times. Yes, having different emotions, with some fluctuation, is normal. But what if our emotional swings go to extremes and become our emotional print? What happens if we become sad, angry, or scared most of the time?

In this case, the body comes out of homeostasis and alters its well-being. Not only the emotional well-being but the physical as well. We can't forget that the body is connected at every level.

Again, what happens when the body says, "Oops, something is wrong with the right engine. Mayday! Mayday!" Similarly, the mind recognizes something is wrong with the body. The right engine is showing fumes and the body needs to adjust as necessary.

In the case of the human body, we need to understand that it's normal to feel sadness at times. What is not normal is depression. It's normal to feel fear. But what's not normal is to have a panic disorder. It is normal to have intrusive thoughts such as, "Did I do this, or did I do that?" But it's not normal to have an increase in obsessive-compulsive disorder (OCD) symptoms. What I mean by not normal is that situations push the body out of homeostasis, like a nose-dive of a twin-engine plane.

Does this mean that when something doesn't feel normal that we need to make it normal? No! We simply want to help our emotional well-being get closer to its baseline. For example, my baseline in the morning is- I wake up, I might be a bit tired but I move into my scheduled day. I begin feeling refreshed after a healthy breakfast, and good about the day's activities. Then I get a call from a friend who gives me some bad news which results in me feeling sad. It's not abnormal for bad news to make us feel sad.

What I'm hoping to encourage people to do from my example, is to "periodically check your emotional baseline." Is the baseline, even with some sadness, normal? If not, notice the imbalance of the homeostasis state. Referencing this chart can help you determine your emotional print.

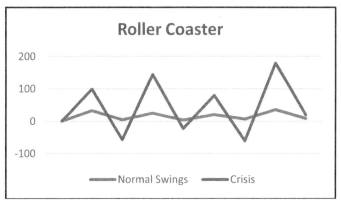

Let's take a deeper look at sadness as an emotional example. When people feel sadness, the brain gets altered causing action of the hypothalamus and pituitary gland. This causes a release of specific hormones that control stress and other functions of the body. The body then senses an imbalance of homeostasis and says, "Oh, something is wrong. I cannot ignore flying with a broken engine. We need to fix this mess." As the body continues to release molecules that cause a state out of homeostasis, it begins damaging certain parts of the body such as blood vessels, muscular structure, and organs. As time goes on, one turns from being a healthy person to someone having issues, imbalances, and breakages in the body, causing sickness and disease.

If this continues, the other engine then has a problem. Like a twin-engine plane, you have two bad engines, then you go down; this is the crisis stage. The body sees crisis and the emotion-body roller coaster begins. At this stage, the mind is affecting the body, and the body is affecting the mind. A person then needs to know how to adjust to the emotional changes of the ups and downs in order to keep the body in a healthy homeostasis state. Continuously connecting with the emotions, a person can ask themselves the following to determine their emotional print.

1) Is the cause of my upset something within my control?
2) Is there anything I can do about my situation at this moment?
3) Is something physical going on in my body that I need to pay attention to?
4) Am I on a roller coaster of emotions, or just a bit upset at the moment?

Sometimes trying to adjust the state of homeostasis repeatedly can get us into what is called "the homeostatic burden." This is the burden of the body trying to forcibly correct itself. This cycle actually increases stress. Emotionally, we start feeling worse over time, rather than better. An organ that is being impacted activates the hypothalamus-pituitary-adrenal (HPA) axis. This sets off a loop, releasing yet other hormones or another kind of signal called the "Northan." This molecule induces even more and more unhappiness and restlessness. And on and on the cycle goes, as shown below.

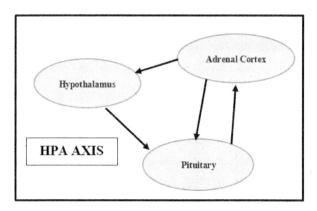

In this situation the body says, "Right now there is no time for emotional well-being. I am going to increase the dysphoria." This causes the opposite state of euphoria. What the body really needs to do is break the unhealthy cycle. Memory and recall become a problem as the mind feels overwhelmed. Confusion sets in, and the body suffers exhaustion. When the mind gets disturbed, the body becomes disturbed. When the body gets disturbed, the mind suffers as well. The emotion-body roller coaster goes round and round, up and down.

When it seems unlikely that the body will regulate, it moves into a state of "allostasis"- a situation where the body begins adapting by reducing the functions of certain organs. At this point the body just cannot continue struggling to find homeostasis with an unregulated emotional environment. The body simple adapts to the cycle. This is the point when the disease or imbalance turns to chronic illness. The immune system, nervous system, and endocrine system are all impacted. Even worse than all this, the architecture of the brain begins to change.

Anyone familiar with brain diagnosis or with experience of panic disorder can identify with this. A lot of changes happen to the body, signaled by the brain, on the physical, mental, and emotion planes. This is the roller coaster. It can be unstoppable and is not fun for anyone. It is also the time when pain sets in. It is not only emotional pain, but pain in the hip, in the heart, in the gut; it can be anywhere in the body. Then the ability to walk upstairs or have any kind of fun seems impossible. What can bring a person out of this challenging cycle?

Let's start with these steps.

1) Be aware of fluctuating emotions.
2) Gather as much emotional awareness as possible.
3) Focus on the internal psychosis.
4) Determine if the stress is real or perceived.
5) Determine what specifically is causing the stress, being as precise as possible.
6) Is an old belief rearing its ugly head? If so, name it.
7) Is there a value issue involved in the stress? If so, name it.
8) NAME- Realize and Identify.
9) CLAIM- Personal Responsibility.
10) AIM- For a lifestyle medicine approach to healing.

I will break this down into a three-part model for a recovery plan of the emotion-body roller coaster, from allostasis into a state of ease. The three parts involve: the healthcare practitioner, the individual, and the support system of the individual.

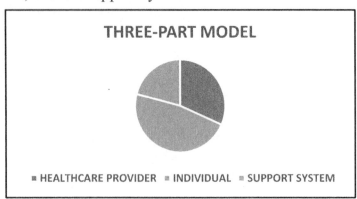

1) Healthcare practitioner
   ➢ Understand the need to slow the roller coaster down.

- ➤ Treat the person as a whole being- mind, body, and spirit.
- ➤ Have methods to stop the cycle.
- ➤ Identify tools to address the emotional body, as well as the physical symptoms.
- ➤ Educate on Lifestyle Medicine.
  - o Identify - Intelligence Quotient (IQ) and Emotional Quotient (EQ).
  - o Place a focus on the value of nutrition.
  - o Identify support systems with clients/patients.
  - o Discuss spiritual matters and issues.
  - o Discuss the importance of outdoor activities and exercise.
  - o Assess passions, interests, and hobbies.
- ➤ Build a support team of holistic practitioner and specialists with intervention protocols:
  - o Additional coaches or psychotherapists
  - o Healing modality specialists
  - o Body care workers- chiropractor, acupuncture, massage therapist
2. The individual- client/patient
- ➤ Be sure they will take full responsibility for their health.
  - o Recognize and understand the necessary emotional environment.
  - o Have a willingness to learn about Lifestyle Prescriptions® Medicine.
  - o Identify personal social support systems.
    - ▪ Be assured it is okay to ask for help.
  - o Work on forgiveness of all grudges that have been held for long and short time periods.
  - o Recognize the personal emotional footprint.
    - ▪ Identify the differences between the states of sadness and depression.

- Discover if they are a person sad by nature? (Sometimes traits and attributes that people are born with set them up for a chronic, temperamental sad reaction to life.)
- Have them identify the root of their sadness or depression
- Are they slow or fast by nature in their thinking process? (The book, *Thinking, Fast and Slow*, by Daniel Kahneman, offers a lot of insight into how different thinking processes impact the brain in dealing with emotions, decisions, relationships, and life in general.)
- Have they learned to not react instantaneously to emotions?
- Have they learned to identify where they are on the emotion-body roller coaster?
- Have they learned to identify with their emotions consciously?
- They can ask:
  - Is my emotion normal, abnormal, or extreme?
  - Have I learned to not run away from my emotions?
  - Is there something I can learn from my emotional state in flux?
- Are they open to holistic practitioners and a holistic intervention plan?
- Can they find some joy in daily life and even in small activities?

3. Support system- Helps the person's mind and body to slow down.
   - Identify and enlist their support
     - People who they live with.
     - Coaches, mentors, and friends.
     - Church or other groups.

- o Determine to not push people away who truly love and want to help.
- o Ask for hope, hugs, and prayers.

Working through these steps with each client could draw a greater understanding and conviction to their part in the healing process. It could look something like this (shown below) as a form, as if they are making a contract with you, and ultimately with themself.

As your client, I agree to take responsibility for my health and well-being. Together we have identified some ways I can do this. I choose to be on a path of well-being, not a path of destruction. I am ready to make changes in my life, beginning with some small steps.

I am ready, willing, and able to work with you as my mentor to:

- ➤ Coach me through some milestones
- ➤ Break down big goals into smaller, achievable objectives.
- ➤ Help empower me in achieving goals.
- ➤ Help me make sense out of how and what I feel. This will help me move on to the next milestone.
- ➤ Learn the Lifestyle Medicine and Lifestyle Prescriptions® approach to health and healing.

My part to recovery and healing.	Initial
1. Recognize and understand the necessary emotional environment I need to be in.	
2. Have a willingness to learn about Lifestyle Prescriptions® Medicine.	

3. Identify my personal support system and ask them for help.	
4. Work on forgiving all grudges that I've held for short periods of time or for a lifetime.	
5. Be conscious of my emotional footprint, recognizing when I am feeling sadness or depression, why, and where it came from.	
6. Determine if it is my nature to think slow or fast. (Everyone has their own style of thinking that impacts their emotions and resolutions.)	
7. Work on not reacting instantaneously to my emotions.	
8. Strive to consciously identify where I am on the emotion-body roller coaster.	
9. When I am feeling emotional, I will ask myself, "Is there something I can learn from my emotional reaction to this situation?"	
10. I am open to holistic practitioners and a holistic intervention plan.	
11. I will find joy in daily life and small activities throughout each day.	

CLIENT SIGNATURE:_____

DATE:_____

In summary, our mind and body are on a continuous roller coaster. If the roller coaster is too cyclical, our body hits a crisis-mode which is the allostatic state.

At this point our organs can begin to malfunction, and chronic disease ensues. This is a signal to be aware of what's happening in the internal psyche. If we adopt this three-part model, I truly believe a lot of people would have fewer chronic illnesses, and faster solutions with disease.

The key to healing chronic disease is a mindset that consciously stays aware of the emotion-body roller coaster syndrome.

Chapter Sixteen

Jane Oelke ND, Ph.D. - Fibromyalgia, Chronic Pain, Emotions, and Limiting Beliefs

Jane Oelke ND, Ph.D., Lifestyle Prescriptions® Health Coach Specialist (LPHCS) is a certified Naturopath- Doctor of Homeopathy with more than 28 years of experience in natural energy techniques and functional medicine, specializing in helping clients find the root cause of their symptoms. ↗ naturalchoicesforyou.com

When talking about limiting beliefs and trapped emotions affecting the pain healing response, a few questions come to mind:

- What triggered the event?
- Why wasn't there complete healing after an injury or trauma?

I often see psychological conflicts that are stored in organ tissues. They are usually triggered by:

- A traumatic event
- Ongoing stressful activities

This leads to:

- Chronic issues
- Daily reoccurring thoughts
- Ongoing stress triggers

The reoccurring thoughts:

- Hold negative patterns in the body
- Prevent healing

Creating awareness of triggers is the only way out of pain:

- Become consciously aware of triggers.
- Become aware of emotions and limiting beliefs.

Chronic pain becomes a message of stuck energy in our body:

- The low energy metabolism affects the body's ability to move energy.
- This lowers mitochondria's ability to function properly.

About 25,000 mitochondria in each muscle cell create energy in our bodies.

- Proper functioning cells lead to health.
- Poorly functioning cells cause hypersensitivity to pain.

Hypersensitivity to pain, hyperalgesia:

- Specifically affects a neurotransmitter- gamma-aminobutyric acid (GABA).
- A sign of this is sensitivity to noise.

GABA:

- A natural chemical produced by the brain.
- Is an inhibitor of an overreaction to pain, smells, and noise.

Pain is one of the most common ailments that people become hypersensitive to, especially with fibromyalgia. I believe:

- Chronic pain is the result of stuck energy in the body.
- Pain needs to move out of the body for relief and healing.

Pain can result anywhere in the body from:

- An injury.
- A traumatic event or experience.

Trauma:

- Leads to inflammation.
- Inflammation prevents complete healing.

When stress continues for too long:

- The body can't support complete healing.
- A chronic pain cycle begins from metabolic imbalances.

Stress from reoccurring pain and related thoughts hurt:

- Emotions and limiting beliefs from metabolic upset.
- Tissues in the body that store emotions.

Walk through this with me. This is an encounter that I had with a client. Jane had been suffering from chronic back pain for a few weeks.

Jane, "I have chronic pain and doctors can't figure out the cause or what to do about it. I've been to a doctor and chiropractor. I've taken Tylenol and other medications, and absolutely nothing is relieving this constant pain."

I asked her, "When exactly do you remember the pain starting?"

Jane, "It was probably four weeks ago. I woke up on a Sunday morning. I remember waking up with back pain but with no reason for it."

I asked her what happened on the Saturday night before. After she thought about it, she said, "Well, I was out with my husband for dinner, and we had an argument. I forgot all about that until now."

I asked if the argument had been resolved. At first, she said, "I think so." Then recanted, "Maybe not since it is still heavy on my mind."

This is a prime example of holding emotions in the body.

If we could take any emotional pain and hold it in our hands for a long time, we will feel the pain eventually cramping our fingers, then our hands, then even up to our arms. After twenty minutes or so, opening the hands and shaking them off, you will notice the cramping subside. This is the same thing that happens throughout the body when holding emotional pain.

Not very surprising to me, Jane called me the day after our meeting and reported, "The pain is gone!"

Let's look at the anatomy of this and how trapped emotions relate to the tissues in the body.

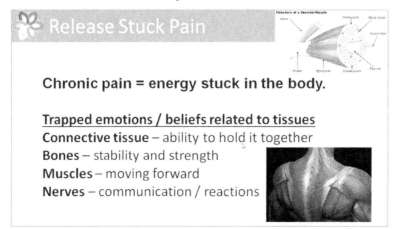

Look at the connective tissue in the block above. Connective tissue, bones, blood vessels, and even cartilage, are all made of collagen. Collagen acts like an intracellular glue providing support to the whole body. How well we are holding our life together is shown in our collective tissues. A proper balance of collagen helps the body function painlessly, an improper or lack of collagen will cause chronic pain and weakness throughout the body.

Relate the function of collagen to your bones. They provide stability and strength. A lack of collagen can cause a breakdown of cartilage, and the covering of the bones, thus causing inflammation. This is medically known as arthritic pain and causes arthritic-type symptoms causing stiffness, aches, and pain throughout the body. This is all related to the stability and strength in the body as well as in life. Our muscles represent our ability to "move forward." Anyone with arthritis could ask themself, "How capable am I of moving forward- physically and emotionally?"

I work with a lot of clients suffering from fibromyalgia. "Fibro"- fiber; "Myalgia" – muscle pain. Fiber + Chronic Muscle Pain = Fiber-Myalgia = Pain in the fibers. Fibromyalgia usually begins after some type of trauma or upsetting event and is characterized by:

- Widespread musculoskeletal pain
- Fatigue after hours of sleep
- Memory issues
- Mood swings
- Digestive issues

Fibromyalgia is symptomatically diagnosed, based on symptoms only, and is known as a syndrome. It affects muscles throughout the whole body, almost like a "brain freeze" to the muscles. Relating the emotions to the body, we could ask a person, "Are you feeling difficulty moving forward in your life?" Or, to get a little deeper into the mind-body connection, "How are your muscles and nerves feeling?" The nerves are the communication vessels to the muscles throughout the body. Radiating nerve pain, pinched nerves, or this type of pain, will cause reactions within the body and prevent the healing process.

To help identify the root cause of the emotional issue, which results in physical pain, we need to look for a key event or trigger.

It always relates to trapped emotions which can come from any number of situations.

Let's look at a few:

- Thoughts of self-worth and value.
  - o Can show up from emotions of guilt, shame, or sadness.
  - o Relates to muscles, and feelings of being unappreciated, undervalued or rejected.
  - o Very prevalent in people suffering from fibromyalgia.
- Paralyzing trauma.
  - o Social pressures from others cause muscles to become almost paralyzed.
  - o Affects nerves and muscles.
  - o Causes nerve pain.
  - o Relates to feelings of fear and helplessness.
  - o Causes difficulty in moving forward with social relationships.

I'd like to share another client encounter with you. We'll call her Ann. Ann told me that she was at work one day, and someone that she didn't usually work with came into her office. She turned towards him by twisting her neck, and he told her some bad news about one of her family members. Without realizing it at the time, this trauma affected Ann's neck. Every time she turned her neck after that, her neck would start hurting. She was holding trauma in the nerves of her neck, which caused a pinched nerve, and related pain. We can see how recognized, as well as unrecognized, traumas can affect the ability to heal. These traumas affect our energy and ability to let go of painful issues, making it harder or even impossible to recover.

Another aspect to look at with fibromyalgia is survival issues. These past traumas can cause the inability to "digest" previous events that affect the fascia. Fascia is the communication avenue to the muscles. Fascia trauma comes from anger and conflict and is usually stored in the lower back. Many pain relief studies look at the lower back as a common area of unresolved conflicts dealing with anger and resentment. As these conflicts are stressful at the time of an event, we often don't want to deal with them at the moment. These stress events become unconsciously held in our tissues and released later when the stress level lowers. We essentially forget to resolve the issue, or purposely or subconsciously bury it, creating trapped emotions and eventually leading to limiting beliefs.

I did a research project a couple of years ago where I asked 45 people their thoughts and beliefs about their nerve pain damage and possible related beliefs. The most common responses were, "I am not strong enough to deal with the stress in my life." In another word, "I'm not holding my life together very well." The other, "I have too many responsibilities." This belief relates to the self-worth issues held in the connective tissues.

I've seen young mothers with fibromyalgia trying to balance care for their children and extended families, looking after their homes, and wanting to be responsible community members, all while neglecting themselves. People in this situation or others with a strong sense of responsibility for others need to figure out how to take care of themselves. If we work with people to help them release blocked emotions and beliefs, so many people can be helped and relieved of their chronic pain.

Let's look at some steps that could help towards this end goal of releasing negative and blocked emotions and beliefs. These steps could provide a walk-through with clients, from realization to healing.

1) Increase awareness of the mind-body connection.
2) Pay attention to self-talk patterns and habits.
3) Seek a connection between the pain and a situation, event, or trauma.

4) Take time to understand how emotions, beliefs, self-talk, and pain, affect your life.
5) Listen for hidden perceptions that identify programs running constantly through your mind. Many are like computer loops that keep circling back, around and around.
6) Notice how much time you talk about and verbalize your pain. This helps hold it in the tissues.
7) Look at pain as a signal from the body. There is always a message in pain.
8) Be curious about symptoms, don't just try and suppress them.
9) Consciously be aware of how tightly you hold on to personal beliefs.
10) The longer the pain and situation continue, the more solid the belief systems become in the body, thus continuing to worsen the pain.

Healing becomes chronic with attachment to negative triggers and patterns.

Staying in chronic negative patterns suppresses healing. It prevents any forward movement. Emotions and beliefs come from perceptions and attachments to them. With conscious awareness and a desire for healing comes inner freedom to evaluate painful experiences. A self-evaluation for clients could look something like this:

1) Can something be learned from the experience of pain?
2) Can a new story about pain shift beliefs and perspectives?
3) Shifting internal beliefs, programs, and triggers, can break stuck energy, and allow for healing.
4) Visualize and create new stories of how you want to feel and what you want, taking your attention away from what you don't want.

5) Understand what it means to live in the present moment, versus in the past. In the present moment is joy; in the past is pain.
6) Pay attention to negative cycles that can be broken.
7) Incorporate physical movement, activity, and exercise, into every day.
8) Learn to smile about little things.
9) Practice some breathing techniques. Inhale fresh air, exhale the pain.
10) Stay hydrated. A lack of water has more of a negative impact on the body than most can even imagine.
11) Realize that some small changes in your health habits can make big differences in your life.
12) Increase your sense of internal control by acting intentionally.
13) Change perceptions to the stories you tell yourself.
14) Stop covering up the pain with medication. This never works long-term. Suppressing symptoms won't make positive or permanent changes in your life.
15) Working with a Lifestyle Medicine health coach can help a person understand and reflect on personal experiences, and act on new insights.
  ➢ Lifestyle Medicine health coaches:
    • Help clients become aware of their belief systems and patterns.
    • Help with "reframing" to create new pain reactions.
    • Listen and hear without judgment.
    • Help build resilience to life challenges.
    • Help with goal setting and moving forward.
    • Identify blind spots and barriers that others can't see.
    • Create lasting change.

Fibromyalgia is not a single disease; it's a syndrome. A syndrome is a complex array of different symptoms that are going on in the body. There are no known viruses connected with fibromyalgia. But low energy metabolism has been identified. And it's this low energy from the mitochondria in the muscles that causes fatigue. Mitochondria are the energy cells in our body. And the adult human body has about ten million billion of these.

One way to heal is to improve the functioning of the mitochondria by creating more energy in the body. We do this mostly by eating well and providing healthy nutrition to cells. Avoiding processed food is as important. And staying active is vital to keeping energies moving. Staying hydrated, breathing, sleeping well, and relaxing, are also important to any type of healing effort.

Other aspects of health that are important to look at with fibromyalgia are:

- Diet
- Toxins in the body
- Survival issues and related beliefs
- Hormone balances and imbalances
- The immune system
- Digestive issues:
  - o Can cause bloating or heartburn.
  - o Impact the body's ability to digest nutrients.
  - o Can worsen with financial worries.
  - o Can impact a host of organs.
  - o Cause congestion throughout the body.
  - o Are related to chronic sinus infections.

I have helped resolve fibromyalgia with many of my clients. I use different Lifestyle Medicine techniques to help them understand different aspects of both illness and healing. We discuss their digestive issues and the impact it has on health and the immune system. We talk about energy and energy systems in the body. We look at hormones and the importance of a good, balanced system.

When working with a client, I don't just look at one symptom. Someone might come to me with a headache or a digestive issue. I look at the whole body, the big picture. What is going on, and where might the energies be stuck? It's interesting to watch people begin to see and understand the mind-body connection and realize that a headache may not be just caused by one simple factor or even fibromyalgia. It's a whole-body perspective that needs serious investigation.

I have some quizzes that I give to my clients to see if their symptoms are caused by low energy or hormonal imbalance. This quiz also helps determine if their health issues are triggered by toxins or adrenal stress. Adrenal stress is another issue to look at. Stress and anxiety result from holding on to uncomfortable experiences. I often see people with anxiety issues and am asked to help with resolutions. Anxiety is a big issue and relates to a lot of emotions; all need to be addressed.

Shame is another common emotion. Or some people just feel like they are never listened to. These things all need to be explored with the client. The more interaction with a client, the better we can understand the underlying causes of health issues. Beyond listening to just health issues, it's important to listen to what's going on in a person's life. Are they having relationship difficulties? Are they in a job they hate or feel unappreciated in? Do they like where they live? Do they feel safe in their life? Most everyone looks at their health issues as physical. But there is usually an underlying imbalance preventing people from fully healing. Some people don't understand the dynamics of the mind-body connection, while others just feel they don't want to deal with deep emotional issues. Sometimes a lack of healing is a lack of understanding. But surprisingly, sometimes it's because not everyone really wants to get better.

Lifestyle Prescriptions® Medicine offers hope for full healing which is something no other approach does. Beginning treatment with just three micro-habit changes, or "lifestyle prescriptions" can have a profound impact on chronic fibromyalgia pain and a journey back to healing and health.

For simple starters, encourage clients/patients to:

1) Understand the importance of hydration and getting enough water daily.
2) Take time to breathe. Even stopping for just five minutes for some long, deep breathing exercises can make a huge difference in calming internal stress.
3) Be aware of self-talk. Listen to what you say to yourself; it is uplifting or a put-down? Feel how the words impact your body.
4) Pay close attention to each of these three areas listed above. Pay attention to "where" the body is holding pain. See if you can figure out what message the pain might be trying to send.

There is always hope for healing with fibromyalgia. I have seen it myself over and over again. A person needs the will to recover which is most successful with a good coach. Lifestyle Prescriptions® Medicine approach includes:

1) An evidence-based, four-pillar protocol to help clients increase vitality, immunity, and mind-body strength.
2) A ten-step, root-cause analysis to identify triggers, emotions, beliefs, and lifestyle habits, that impact the organ-mind-brain anatomy.

3) Provide root-cause, health coaching with micro-habit change skills.
4) Improve the client's ability to self-heal and auto-regulate.

Chapter Seventeen

Dr. Tom O'Bryan - How Food Choices Determine a Better Way for Your Health

Dr. O'Bryan is considered a "Sherlock Holmes" of chronic disease. He holds teaching faculty positions with the Institute for Functional Medicine and the National University of Health Sciences and has trained tens of thousands of practitioners. ↗ thedr.com

There is a point that most people miss in exploring how they can feel and function better during a health crisis. Many doctors reference this in a roundabout way. I want to do a deep dive into the research on dealing with chronic health issues- such as fibromyalgia, rheumatoid arthritis, lupus, or cognitive decline in Alzheimer's patients.

Blue Cross Blue Shield, one of the largest health insurance companies in the United States reported in a February 2020 Forbes magazine article;

> *"Early-onset dementia and Alzheimer's disease jumped 200% among commercially insured Americans between the ages of 30 and 64 over a recent five-year period."*

And,

> *"The report shows 131,000 people between the ages of 30 and 64 were diagnosed with either form of dementia in 2017. The average age of someone with either condition is 49 and women are disproportionately impacted than men."*

Are you familiar with the term "canary in the coal mine?" For those not familiar with it, it is a term coined back in the late 1800s. Coal miners used to bring caged canaries with them down into the mines. If there was a gas leak of methane or carbon monoxide, the humans couldn't smell it. As a result of any leakage, the canary would stop singing, die, and signal the workers of a leak. This would immediately instigate a mass exit to safety.

The canary was used as a test, not a guess, of a deadly possibility. This same principle can be used in our healthcare. But does testing give us the whole story? A person can be diagnosed with diabetes, told not to eat sugar, and still have issues. The problem might not be the sugar intake but the way the body processes insulin due to toxin chemicals in the body or other reasons.

We can start by looking at the most prevalent pathology of almost all diseases- inflammation. The National Institute of Environmental Health Services (NIH) states:

> *"Inflammation is a normal part of the body's defense to injury or infection, and in this way, it is beneficial. But inflammation is damaging when it occurs in healthy tissues or lasts too long. Known as chronic inflammation, it may persist for months or years."*

It goes on to say, "Chronic inflammatory disease contributes to more than half of the deaths worldwide."

What we learn from this research is that inflammation is a way that the body helps protect us, but to an extreme, it is involved in degenerative diseases. The Center for Disease Control (CDC) reports that inflammation is a factor in eight out of ten leading causes of death. Inflammation seems tied to the weakest link in the body- be it the kidneys, heart, brain, liver, breast, or any part of the body, possibly one damaged in an accident that has become weakened or compromised.

We should all be asking, "How do we begin reducing inflammation in the body?" The answer is, "Take care of the gut microbiome." This is the environment of the gut that modulates. This means it has a controlling influence over all other parts. Because of this, it's important to know how to build a healthy microbiome. The only thing more important than this is staying hydrated with a half-ounce of water per pound of body weight per day. The importance of the water intake is to continually flush accumulating toxins from the body.

Medical research shows relationships between systemic chronic inflammation as shown below in Chart #1.

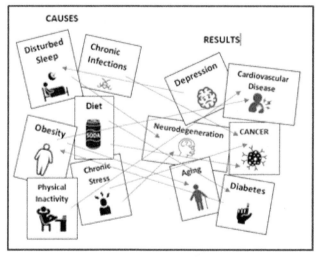

Note the relationships between causes and results. You can see the mechanism at the core of practically all chronic diseases, that all things in the body are related. Rather than recognizing and understanding the relationships, people just want a pill for the symptoms; they just want to feel better, and "Now!" Pills are pointless for long-term healing. You need to address the cause of the inflammation. Chronic inflammation is fuel to the fire, but not the fire itself. The patient's top priority is feeling better. The job or priority of healthcare providers should be to look for the source of the inflammation, which is rarely one cause. As accrued poisonous compounds originating from cigarette smoke cause various health conditions, and so do many toxins originating from day-to-day exposures as they accumulate in the body. Any combination of habits can cause a multitude of health problems.

When I discuss this with doctors, they tell me it makes sense; yet is something they hadn't thought about before. I explain these conditions are referred to as sensitivity-related illnesses. (SRI). This refers to adverse clinical states elicited by exposure to low-dose diverse environmental triggers. These could be mold, electromagnetic frequencies, foods such as those containing gluten, synthetics, chemicals, and even inhalants like pollen and air pollutants. All of these can wear down the body's immune system over time and cause several chronic issues. Under these conditions, the immune system kicks in to help protect the body, causing an inflammatory response. It can manifest in the joints and be medically diagnosed as rheumatoid arthritis, as a skin issue diagnosed as psoriasis, or in the nerves with a diagnosis of multiple sclerosis. It is always the root cause that needs to be identified. This is the basis of Lifestyle Prescriptions® University training. Without root cause analysis, long-term healing is nearly impossible.

When a person's toxic load reaches a threshold, the immune system provokes a low-grade systemic chronic inflammatory response. This creates cytokines to kill whatever it identifies as the invader. At this point of hitting the threshold, there is cognitive decline such as Alzheimer's, Parkinson's, multiple sclerosis (MS), or vitiligo. It doesn't matter which medical diagnosis a person is labeled with; the core mechanism still needs to be identified.

This hypersensitivity state responds to any negative exposures creating a storm of inflammation that accrues in the body.

Chronic inflammation kills off tissue and creates a host of symptoms. This is called multi-morbidity, simply meaning, there are two or more health conditions needing consideration.

We can relate this to alcohol abuse and the relationship between liver disease and cardiomyopathy. Stomach cancer, osteoporosis, brain issues, and nervous system disorders, all can result from long-term alcohol consumption. It is only when you apply appropriate interventions, meaning you make changes and get rid of the triggers, that recovery and healing can take place.

I want to show you the mechanism that sets the stage for all inflammatory issues. First, I want to introduce you to my friend and mentor, Alessio Fasano. Fasano is a Professor of Nutrition at the Harvard School of Public Health, as well as the Chief of Pediatric Gastroenterology and Director of the Celeriac Research Center, at Massachusetts General Hospital, a Harvard Medical School.

He and his team, at the University of Maryland School of Medicine, were the first to identify the leaky gut syndrome. It was in 2000, and ever since then, he has been publishing information about how it contributes to disease. In 2019 he wrote the article *All Disease Begins in the Leaky Gut.* He explained the role of a protein (considered a biomarker of increased intestinal permeability, called Zonulin. Here is where he says all chronic inflammatory disease begins - diabetes, chronic depression, anxiety, and on and on.

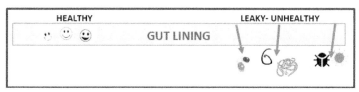

This concept is now being taught at Harvard Medical School. Young doctors now entering this institution are receiving a modernized education that teaches about the leaky gut syndrome. Doctors graduating in the past are only able to receive this training postgraduate.

Regardless of whatever health condition is causing inflammation, the gut is playing a role. This is the core of activation for the immune system.

In Professor Fasano's article, he describes the perfect storm in the development of all chronic diseases. Most patients arrive at doctor visits with a list of symptoms and are sometimes even barely able to function. You can go through the five components of the perfect storm with each patient. Let's look at them here:

1) Genetics - Can we do anything about genetics? Can we turn genes off and on? We show clients that the answer to these questions is "yes." Research shows that with the proper diet and lifestyle we can enhance our gene makeup.
2) Environmental triggers
   - What we eat- foods
   - What we drink- Toxic water and sugar-filled soda drinks
   - What we breathe- toxic air indoors and outside
   - Mold- causes inflammation and deterioration in the brain
3) Dysbiosis, a microflora imbalance causing inflammation
4) Leaky gut - Imagine your gut as a 20-foot-long tube winding around inside of you. Then it blows a gasket and springs a leak. Gut contents leak to other parts including the bloodstream. (As shown in Chart #2)
5) Immune response - Activates to fight an intruder, creating inflammation in the bloodstream and throughout the body.

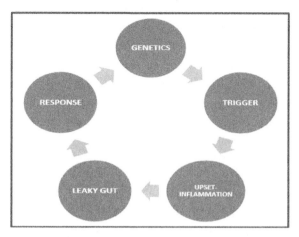

As we can see, inflammation continues throughout the body once this cycle begins. Then depending on the body's weakest point, the system begins to break down into multiple issues and symptoms. The perfect storm. In any case, the cause of the inflammation in the body needs to be identified. This is the three-step process to look at breaking this vicious and harmful cycle.

REMOVE, REBUILD, REPAIR

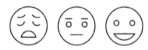

1) REMOVE environmental exposers
2) REBUILD the microbiome from unhealthy to healthy
3) REPAIR leaky gut by changing the microbiome

When we learn to reduce inflammation in the body, we become healthier. Our bodies are designed to work this way; we are meant to age gracefully. Inflammation anywhere in the body breaks down cells causing faster aging and unhealthy situations. We need to always remember that the cause of inflammatory issues is what needs to be addressed with any chronic health problem.

With an understanding of the leaky gut syndrome, I want to challenge doctors to look at all health issues from a different perspective. I urge you to work with patients in helping them experience what true wellness feels like. If a person wants to boost their immunity, lose weight, rid themself of chronic disease, or address new health issues before they turn chronic, then address leaky gut syndrome. The successful process I've developed with thousands of people in this three-step process is simply- to remove, rebuild, and repair.

Life is too short to feel anything but energized and comfortable in the body.

A leaky gut can wreak havoc on nutrient absorption, memory, and energy. By healing the digestive system, you awaken energy, improve mood and focus, and increase assimilation of nutrients.

Follow your gut to the body's natural ability to heal within a supportive environment for positive and permanent changes.

Chapter Eighteen

Louise Harris - Helping Children and Families with Neurological Disorders, Anxiety, and Sleep Issues

Louise Harris is a Researcher, Educator, and Health Coach specializing in Neurological Disorders. She is also the Founder of Coming Alive, a Natural Health and Well-being Practice in the United Kingdom. ↗ comingalive.co.uk

The problem that families face with children having neurological issues, anxiety, or sleep issues, is often that they are given a label. Parents simply accept this, and they have little help in understanding their children's challenges. Apart from sometimes being offered medications or given a strategy, they are often on their own. Some feel helpless and scared, and even worried for their children's futures.

I'm going to share a story about a family that I know very well, and their little boy named Remo. He was born slightly earlier than expected. He had a floppy larynx and went blue at six weeks old. He had a lot of gut issues, constipation, reflux, and colic, and was not the most pleasant baby. He struggled to sleep and struggled with milk or anything else offered to him. When he turned two, he become even more finicky, with people saying, "He is acting out those terrible twos." Not acknowledging a difference from other two-year-old, his mother convinced herself he was just acting normal for his young age.

When Remo started school, he was instantly labeled a bully for bumping into people with no spatial awareness of things around him. He struggled through school and challenged his teachers who felt his behavior was just careless. Without any support with his struggles, Remo began experiencing anxiety issues. His internal stress continued to the point of him picking his fingers raw to the bone. He was "picking his way through his anxiety." His mother finally decided to move him to another school. Knowing that Remo didn't learn as most other children she looked for a school that would accommodate and understand her son's struggles and distinct learning style. Through caring observation, his mother noticed Remo needed more processing time when asked a question. His teachers saw this as abnormal behavior or that he was being rude. But his mother recognized it as a learning style. Some people's brains just operate with needing more processing time. Best-selling author Daniel Kahneman refers to this as "slow thinking", and not being good or bad, right or wrong, just individualized.

Remo's mother finally felt some support and relief in helping her son when she began working with a Special Educational Needs Coordinator (SENCo) and having her son properly diagnosed. These SENCO specialist teachers are trained in working with children who don't fit into the mold of "normality." They are trained to understand children with special or additional needs and learning requirements. After years of misdiagnoses and misunderstandings of Remo's learning issues, there was finally some relief and help.

What are the main areas of need for students with SEN?

The code of practice has identified **four** major areas of need for students with **SEN**:

- Learning and <u>cognition</u>;
- Interaction and <u>Communication</u>;
- Social, Emotional and Mental Health;
- Physical and <u>Sensory</u>;

Remo's mother continued investigating ways to support her son and considering the causes of his inconsistent stress reactions. Some days he seemed to deal with stress well, other times his anxiety and anger could be extreme. She made it her mission to study and research until she came to answers and solutions. Her hours, months, and years of investigating brought her to a gut-brain connection that could be identified through a hair tissue mineral analysis. This type of testing identifies mineral imbalances, nutritional deficiencies, and ways to correct situations going on in the body that can manifest as learning disabilities and coping struggles

A year and a half into a good treatment program, Remo functioned completely differently.

His anger issues dwindled, his brain seemed to function better and more consistently, and his dyspraxia (developmental coordination disorder) vanished. He was no longer accused of having attention deficit hyperactivity disorder (ADHD). He quit walking into people and objects. And his abilities to read and write improved tremendously even in spite of the fact that teachers earlier had told him he would never learn basic skills.

Watching this amazing transition in her son gave this mother a lot of empathy for other families in this same situation. She was aware of many other children battling labels, bullied by teachers and peers, and struggling to get through life day-to-day.

This is my journey with my son Nathan. The changes and transformations my son Nathan went through with my discoveries were astonishing. At one point Nathan asked me, "Mummy, do you think people in prison might have what I had?" He was able to look back and acknowledge that he had uncontrollable anger issues with an inability to process emotions correctly. This propelled me into a continued study of how I could help other children.

I began setting up a research study, working with children having a lot of different labels. How about this for a list-dyslexia, dyspraxia, dyscalculia, dysgraphia, ADHD, sensory processing disorder (SPD), anxiety, allergy, sleep disorder, developmentally challenged, learning delayed, auditory processing disorder, and on and on. Many people came forward wanting help with their children. I was doing this research all on my own and felt isolated. I was also astonished by the number of parents and children going through the same struggles that my family endured.

We started the study with 62 participants. Of the group, 85% had identified gut issues from a young age, including-constipation, reflux, allergies, and eczema. After hair mineral analysis we discovered that 95% had heavy metal toxicity high enough to cause damage to their bodies and brains. We found these as common symptoms in our test group:

- Headaches
- Daytime drowsiness
- Seizures
- Brain and nerve damage
- Skin problems
- Gut issues
- Flu symptoms and illnesses
- Low iron levels

We also found that with mercury toxicity, there are symptoms of:

- Muscle aches and pains
- Body weaknesses
- Lung and respiratory issues
- Kidney abnormalities
- Chest tightness
- Extreme concentration challenges

A copper imbalance, which was 60% of our test group, showed symptoms of:

- ADD and ADHD
- Anger issues including extreme rage
- Anxiety
- Chronic constipation
- Fatigue
- Insomnia
- Seizures
- Candida and other yeast overgrowths
- Obsessive-compulsive disorder (OCD)

Our testing showed 83% with an out-of-balance sodium-potassium ratio, which negatively impacts the body in these ways:

- Kidney and liver dysfunction
- Adrenal exhaustion
- Digestive issues
- Inflammation

All of our test participants followed our program beginning with a hair tissue mineral analysis. This shows the heavy metal toxicities that didn't necessarily show on other tests. Some people additional had stool testing, urinalysis, or blood work done.

Our testing found that 95% of the participants had heavy metal toxicity at levels impacting their gut and brain. We also discovered through our research that the impact of heavy metals on the gut caused the leaky gut syndrome. As long as there are heavy metals in the gut, it will never heal. The leaky gut provides a breeding ground for bacteria, parasites, yeast, mold, and other destructive pathogens. We also want to note that stress always compounds an unhealthy situation. Removing stress from children's lives is vital to their health and well-being.

Also, removing foods that aggravate the gut is important.

Most people eat these foods daily, which are extremely harmful to the whole gut microbiome.

- Processed foods and sugars
- Corn syrup and sugars
- Gluten
- White starchy pasta
- Potatoes and other inflammatory foods

All these foods cause glucose in the gut which affects the gut-brain signal. Most importantly is not consuming these damaging foods first thing in the morning. This fuels and feeds the gut for the day. This feeds the pathogens and bacteria, beginning the process of irritation and inflammation, and sets up the day or a lifetime for a struggle.

I advocate blueberries as we know the benefits, they provide to brain health. Blended with ground flaxseeds and spinach gives a high omega-3 hit to the body. Coconut milk can also be added for extra health and nutrition. First thing in the morning, this is a very refreshing meal. And replacing sugary and glyphosate-loaded cereals with fresh, healthy foods can make all the difference in the world.

As part of Step 1, the removing phase, in working with children, I encourage parents not to reward children with sugary sweets. I used to do this, so I understand it. But after going through my training and work with Lifestyle Prescriptions® Medicine I see how destructive this is. You can see the devastating cycle on the human body in the chart below. (Chart #1) Ditch the processed foods, the sugar, and the gluten, because all these inflammatory foods are going to affect the way the guts send signals to the brain.

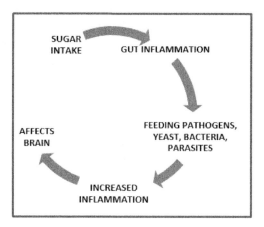

We live in a highly toxic world full of pesticides, herbicides, and insecticides. We need to develop ways to identify, avoid, and remove these sources of toxins.

- Identify sources of pesticides in the environment, in the water we drink and use, and in foods, which could unfortunately even include those marketing as "organic."
- Avoid processed foods, sugars, and glutens.
- Avoid inflammatory foods like:
  o Hydrogenated oils
  o Sports drinks
  o Saturated and trans fats
  o Milk
  o Fried foods
  o Processed meats
  o Alcohol in high amounts
  o Refined carbohydrates
  o Artificial sweeteners
  o Preservatives and artificial colorings
  o Nightshade vegetables- potatoes, tomatoes, eggplant, bell peppers, hot peppers, and paprika

I like encouraging people to look at the Rainbow Diet as a substitute to the processed foods most people are accustomed to eating. The variety of food are colorful fruits and vegetables of red, orange, yellow, green, and purple. This health-positive diet urges adding colorful plant foods to your meals rather than focusing on what not to eat.

Red	apple, cherries, cranberries, pink grapefruit, pomegranate, raspberries, red plums, strawberries, watermelon, beets, red cabbage, red onions
Orange	apricots, cantaloupe, mango, oranges, papaya, peach, carrots, pumpkin, sweet potatoes, yams
Yellow	Asian pears, bananas, lemons, pineapple, starfruit, chickpeas, ginger, lentils, yellow onions, butternut, acorn squash
Green	green grapes, kiwi, limes, green olives, pears, artichokes, avocado, broccoli, cabbage, celery, green beans, peas, kale, spinach, okra
Purple	blackberries, blueberries, figs, plums, purple grapes, prunes, raisins, purple carrots, purple kale, turnips

After the "removing" phase we next work on rebalancing the body by:

- Rebalancing minerals (based on hair mineral analysis testing)
- Helping the body recover from stress and trauma
- Adjusting diet, nutrition, and lifestyle

It is during this time that we start to see huge improvements in the children.

In the next phase – rebalancing, we find that our efforts get a little more challenging. Rebalancing the gut microbiome to a strong and healthy one is necessary. A proper balance of good bacteria is essential to supporting the removal of pathogens and yeast. Here is where we need to retrain reflexes. Everyone is born with reflexes, but some don't integrate until after age three. This can affect the digestive system, the way the brain works, the inflammatory response, and the left brain-right brain connection. With heavy metal toxicity, this all becomes complicated.

One little girl in our first research study had absent seizures with dyslexia and was labeled possibly autistic. She was on epilepsy medication. With our helpful diagnoses and treatment, she is now doing much better in school. I think parents are offered hope when they learn to understand, influence, and have a positive impact on their children's lives. This is what my three-fold process aims to do by removing toxins, rebalancing the mind and body, and restoring vitality to life.

Another important aspect when working with challenged children is to offer a little kindness whenever we can.

They respond well to this as well as needing it. Calmness, love, and empathy work wonders on their psyches. This can help in building some confidence and rebalancing their emotional well-being and internal stress triggers. Reducing stress can calm the nervous system and allow the body to regenerate cells and heal the body from within. Imagine a calm, and not so calm nervous system, like an electrical circuit in the body. Which would you think would be better for a child- a calm frequency, or a frazzled one?

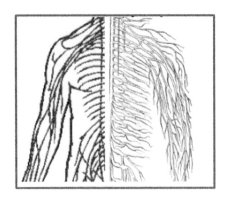

I would love to someday campaign for children with heavy metal toxicity and neurological damage to have time away from school for stress reduction. This would allow their bodies to heal. Like children with cancer are allowed time off school for therapy and treatment, so too should other children who would benefit from a restful, healing period. Children with their minds and bodies already compromised, then stressed more, have little time and energy for healing. The lockdown of 2020 was a beautiful time for so many families given the opportunity to rest, rebalance, and heal.

What I also like to do in working with families is to offer hope. When I am introduced to a new family and the conversation starts like this, I am infuriated, "Hello. This is my child. They are autistic." It comes across as, "My child has this issue or label, and there's nothing I can do about it." In these cases, I don't promise a cure, but I do like to offer hope. I fully believe there is always hope, be it a 10, 20, or maybe even a 100% improvement possibility.

Tips I like to share with parents are:

1) Be verbally supportive. I recommend reassuring phrases with children like, "I understand that you're trying your best." I offer comforting hugs rather than scolding. And I

practice patience and empathy which produces better results than a short-fuse and a strong, heavy tone.

2) As I've mentioned earlier, removing processed foods, junk foods, sugars, white pasta, and bread is of utmost importance to spark a change. These foods end up as glucose in the gut, inflame the gut, and cause a host of unhealthy issues.

3) Identify and remove toxins from inside the home. Quit using toxic cleaners and chemicals and use air purifiers. This is a big step in changing air quality for the most common location of children that parents have some control over.

4) Identify and remove stress from the child's environment, as much as possible.

Realize that working through health issues will involve some costs. There is not only a financial commitment to working with children's health issues but also time commitments. Both time and money are more of investments than painful costs. The benefits are not only to your child but also to others around them, society, and the future. It's a very good investment. When given a shot at it, give it your best.

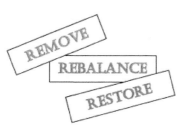

Chapter Nineteen

Bernie Siegel MD - Stories of Wisdom. Healthcare Reimagined

Dr. Siegel is an internationally recognized pioneer in the field of cancer treatment and complementary, holistic medicine. He is the author of the ground-breaking book "Love, Medicine, and Miracles." Bernie will share stories that are entertaining, enlightening, and deeply transformational, from his 50 years of experience with cancer patients. ↗ berniesiegelmd.com

Whenever asked, "How are you?" I often respond in jest with, "I'm depressed. I've run out of my antidepressants and my doctor is on vacation, so I can't refill my prescription." One day when I said this in line at the supermarket, people offered me their pills, asking, "Will this help?" One time I pulled my little prank at the post office only to find a psychiatrist offering me his business card. Laughing at the situation I realized this is not a very good joke in a world with so many depressed people. We all have life-changing experiences of some type, maybe similar to mine.

Another eventful time for me was while attending a conference. I thought it was for doctors, but I discovered after I had gotten there that I was the only physician in the group of 150 people. After speaking, I noticed one of my clients in attendance and asked why she was there. Her reply was, "I like being in your presence. I feel better when I'm around you. And I can't take you home with me after our office visits, so I just wanted to be with you."

Returning to work after that powerful weekend, a Monday morning client said to me, "Bernie, you're changed since we were together last." And he was right, and all simply because of the women's statement that redirected my life. I was able to see the impact that people can have on other people. Caring people can uplift others, and many times with neither party even realizing it.

This epiphany propelled me to start support groups for cancer patients. I began my program with 100 invites. Twelve women showed up to the first gathering including my wife. Curious as to why more people didn't attend, I heard remarks like, "He makes you read books and draw pictures. He talks with you about your feelings. I just don't have time for that." The people that did show up were non-hesitant. They knew when and where to meet and were anxious to get together. This showed me without a doubt who the survivors are, and what type of people can recover from cancer and doctor's death sentences.

I heard a story of one cancer patient in need of cataract surgery. His insurance company refused to cover the cost based on the fact that he had lung cancer and the explanation for no coverage was, "A waste of money." This was very depressing as the man wanted to play with his grandchildren, read the paper, and continue to experience life around him, with or without lung cancer. The man died within a week of being told his surgery would be a waste of money. I'm sure depression played a factor in the situation. I suggested to the family that they sue the insurance company. My observations of insurance company determinations have never been favorable.

I remember the days when the AIDS (acquired immunodeficiency syndrome) epidemic was in full swing. People with the diagnosis were expected to die. Dr. George Solomon's research coined the phrase, "Immune Competent Personality" for those who readily overcome a range of diseases, including AIDS. The key component was the capacity of some to find meaning through stressful life circumstances. I learned from him what could and would make the difference between life and death. I have a resource page on my website with the Immune Competent Personality test.

After a lot of my research, I sent articles to medical journals. The responses were mostly, "Interesting, but not appropriate." It seems that psychiatric professional training separates the person's head from their body. Separating people into pieces and only treating fragments needs to stop. It helps no one.

Here is an example of looking at the body as a whole. One woman I worked with had horrible headaches. I asked her to explain the "feeling" of the pain. She said, "Pressure." I asked if she felt "pressure" in her life. She responded that she did, in her marriage. We discussed looking at this as the cause of her headaches. Another client of mine came to me with cancer. I asked her to describe the "feeling" of her cancer. She said, "It feels like 'failure.' As if my body has failed me." I asked how failure fit into her life? After some thought, she said that her parents both died of suicide when she was young and since then she has felt like a failure.

Some doctors have asked me, "Why do you ask your patients to blame themselves somehow for their illnesses and diseases?"

Many doctors fail to see the correlation between what's going on in one's personal life and emotions, and the impact of that on sickness and chronic disease.

One patient of mine came to see me after being told he was going to die. Since I was close with his family I asked to be told of the funeral. He said he was moving to Colorado to die in the mountains where it is beautiful and peaceful. Not hearing from his family after some time I called the last phone number I had for him. My patient answered the phone. He said he is alive and well in beautiful Colorado.

Then there is the millionaire client of mine who was told he only had a few months to live. When I last saw him, he was dressed poorly. I asked what was up. He said, "When you only have a few months to live, you don't abide by anyone's dress codes." With impending death, his wife convinced him to follow his dream of moving to the sunshine in Miami and spending his days listening to my recordings. I heard years later that he lived his dream in Miami for five and a half years. I've wondered if those who had given him the death sentence know how this story ended? Or thankfully, didn't end as "prescribed."

Next, I want to refer to a man named Aleksandr Solzhenitsyn. Solzhenitsyn was born in Russia in 1918 and is the author of the book *Cancer Ward*. In this novel, he wrote of self-induced healing, which describes spontaneous remission. As a symbol to represent change he used a brightly colored butterfly. And to represent feelings and emotions, he used the rainbow. I strongly believe we need to let the butterfly of change, and emotional growth touch our lives if we are to heal. This book was written as a novel but I find it very non-fictional.

Solzhenitsyn related quite closely to this symbology since he had cancer as well as recovered from it. He felt as if he lived in a cocoon, then busted out, spread his wings, and was off to a new life. He had changed, from being sick to being well.

His representation of the rainbow stood for harmony. Every color represented a different emotion. As life harmonizes, all colors blend into a magical chemistry of one. Written as fiction, but truly non-fiction, I encourage everyone to be inspired by this book.

Another story to share is about an actor student. During a role in a dramatic murder script, some of the actor's blood was taken and tested between acts. The results showed a drop in immune function with elevated stress hormones. The same actor's blood was drawn between acts in a comedy. The exact opposite happened- the immune function rose while the stress hormones lowered. This is just one example I can cite showing laughter having a positive impact on life quality and longevity.

I know of a group of cancer patients who were told to laugh every three hours, even without reason. A control group was told only to laugh when something was funny. At the end of a one-year study, which group do you think had more people alive and well? Laughter therapy is doing wonders as a healing technique for cancer and other chronic diseases.

I had a lot of criticism when I first started leading support groups. Many said to me, "You're not a psychiatrist. You don't even know what you're doing. You could make people feel worse having them talk about their feelings." One psychiatrist was determined to show me wrong. He set up two support groups of women. The control group did not have regular meetings but the other did. The actual "support" group had a better survival rate than the control group. His study failed him, and he became a big advocate of my techniques. Until research like this started happening, I was thought of as nuts.

Another time I had a reporter in my office doing an article about my work. I could sense that she also thought I was a little nutty. I asked her to draw a random picture on a blank piece of paper. She drew a picture of herself with a clock behind her. It only had one hand pointing at the six on the clock. I asked her what happened to her when she was six years old. She said, "I drew the clock because I don't like deadlines." I said, "But there is only one hand on the clock. What happened to you when you were six?" She broke out in tears and told me of sexual and other abuses that happened at that time in her life. This shifted her whole attitude about our interview.

I have so many stories, I could go on forever. I had a patient who had polio when she was young. This caused her a lot of muscle weakness. When she was older, she developed another disease that caused her similar symptoms. She relayed to me that she never liked her body due to what illnesses had done to her. On a positive note, she told me that she didn't want to die hating her body. To shift her feelings about herself she started lying in front of her mirror and telling herself that she loved her body. She said she started with her toes and moved up slowly and systematically up her body. Her adult illness and muscle weakness went into full remission. Do I think this was a coincidence? Certainly not. It was the self-love that healed her.

All these self-healings I am sharing with you are not about preventing death, but rather enjoying life.

I've always believed that love is the best vaccine. A study done at Harvard asked students, "Do your parents love you?" This study revealed that 25% of those who felt loved by their parents developed some type of major illness by midlife. Over 90% of those who didn't feel loved had developed some type of severe illness. To quote someone in the study, "My mother's words were eating away at me and maybe gave me cancer." Her mother constantly belittled her accomplishments and only dressed her in dark colors. We know that up until the age of six, a child's brain wave pattern is similar to that of a hypnotized individual. By the time a child becomes conscious and capable of evaluating their parent's words, they have real struggles on their hands to free themselves from the negative messages most parents have delivered. If we had a "love vaccine" it could help everyone grow up healthier and happier.

I know of a doctor who studied heart attack patients. He noted that if there was a dog in the home, the survival rate was higher than those without a dog. I know from having my own pets what a difference they make in a person's life. They jump up on your lap with their warm, fuzzy love, and your body chemistry changes.

I'd like next to tell you about two different incidents in my office. One is of a cancer client with nine children. She told me she can't die until all of her kids are out of her house and on their own. At this point, her cancer went into remission. After her last child left home cancer returned. I said, "How in the hell can someone control that for twenty years, then let it come back?" I know it was her will that allowed her remission and extended life.

Another client of mine came with his wife and three children. He said, "Since I have cancer and can't work, there is no reason for me to even live." I told him, "Turn your head to the left and I think you'll find four good reasons to live." That statement seemed to knock him out of his negative thinking and woke him up to the importance of relationships and people. I truly believe that when your life has meaning, it keeps the body going and can keep a person alive and well.

I've noticed that a lot of people in hospitals die in the middle of the night. I think this is because doctors aren't there to stop them.

There is an organization and website called Not-On-My-Shift.org. It contains many stories and experiences of ambulance runners keeping people alive with their presence. I've also read an article with the same name, *Not On My Shift*. This was written by three doctors who were proud to keep a critically ill dying man alive. At some point, though they realized they were torturing this man by keeping him alive rather than just letting him die since that's what he wanted to do.

I remember vividly the day my father died. After being bedridden and sick for a while he said to my mother, "Rose, I need to get out of here." He picked a day he wanted to die, a

Sunday afternoon. We had a couple of dozen people over and celebrated his life. With the last visitor, and lots of laughter going on around him, my father drifted off. At the time he didn't know this was the last visitor, but his subconscious did.

And why was he laughing? Because I asked him to recall how he meet my mother. His funny story of meeting her on the beach after losing a coin toss with his guy friends made everyone laugh. Then his ongoing stories of each date after date being a disaster, yet she kept going out with him, how could you help not to laugh? He died laughing with happy memories.

I believe that even after people die, they can continue to communicate with us. My wife died in 2018 and I feel she still communicates with me in many ways. I didn't really believe this until it started happening to me. Bobbie died of a heart attack during the night. I hadn't realized it until I tried to wake her late in the morning. When I touched her body, I had an electrical shock in my heart. Exactly nine months later I had atrial fibrillation. Arriving at the emergency room, I head, "Get him into room 819." They put a wristband on me with the number 8-996633. I noticed all the numbers were adding up to 9s. My wife's birthday was September 9, 9/9. I don't believe any of this was a coincidence. I found comfort in feeling my wife with me during this difficult time. I believe self-induced healing comes through faith, hope, and love.

I had a woman walk into my office one day. My business partner at the time yelled to me, "Bernie, come in here. You're always interested in this stuff." He said the woman had a tumor on her pancreas. She said it was gone and she doesn't feel anything there anymore. I asked her, "What did you do to make a change in your life?" She said, "I left my troubles with God. And oh, what peace it gave me."

Another patient of mine, a landscaper with stomach cancer, had a tumor removed. I told him to have at least one more treatment after surgery to be sure we get rid of all the cancer cells in his lymph nodes. He told me, "It's springtime. I don't have time. I need to focus on my work and make the world a more beautiful place before I die." Six years later my secretary handed me his chart. I told her, "We haven't seen him for six years. He never came back and has likely died by now." She said, "Bernie, open the door." Opening the door, he says to me, "I have a hernia from lifting boulders on a landscaping job." This man was so inspirational over the years that he became like a therapist to me. He constantly pointed out how beautiful life is. We spend time taking walks in the woods and sharing special moments. He lived to be 91 with no signs of returning cancer.

We both loved walking in nature, talking with God, and discussing the mysteries of life. I learned there is a word for this- hisbodedus. This Hebrew word means, "self-solitude"- making time for yourself, meditating. I encourage people to do this every day. It can replace the black and darkness in our life with a rainbow butterfly.

I want to close by remembering the first time Elisabeth Kubler-Ross asked me to draw a picture for her. She followed up with some questions. One, "Why is the number 11 important to you? You drew 11 trees." Her second set of questions was, "Why did you use a white crayon on a white sheet of paper? What are you trying to cover up?"

At the time I was contemplating suicide. Her comments made me feel like I didn't know what to do with my feelings.

I then painted a picture of myself with all my pets and children running away from my house. She asked me, "What are you running away from?"

She asked if I could reframe what I was drawing, seeing, and feeling. I then painted myself as a surgeon with everyone running towards me and into my house.

This self-portrait experience taught me a lot about myself.

I encourage you to do it. Draw a picture of yourself. Put it away for a day, then look at it again. See what can be adjusted and fixed, or "reframed".

Chapter Twenty

Yeliz Ruzgar B.Sc., LPHCS - Life Purpose, Wellness and Longevity (Science of Being)

Yeliz Ruzgar is MANA Life Purpose and Wellness Founder, Lifestyle Prescriptions® University Trainer, Speaker, Author, Licensed Holistic Life Consultant. Yeliz's programs empower people to create a lifestyle that supports their core purpose. She designs individual and group programs to maximize human potential, to attain and sustain optimal life purpose and wellness. ↗ manabook.club

"The two most important days in your life are the day you are born and the day you find out why." – Mark Twain

As the sun was rising on St John's Health Center in Santa Monica, purpose came knocking on her door. There she was, laying on the bed of an emergency room, six doctors around telling her that she needs to go through surgery right away. 'She has a massive, grapefruit-size, bleeding cyst. In rare cases, this can cause death," said one of them. She was confused. She has never been hospitalized before or gone through an operation. Being an immigrant in a foreign country; no family, uncertainty of finances, and all relationships. She didn't know what to do.

Feeling in despair as the doctors were rushing her to make a decision, a voice within whispered:

"Let's heal this together and help others to heal from within. This cyst can be removed with this operation, or you can also go through hormonal therapy with prescribed pills but it may come back if you don't treat the root cause. You are treating only the effect with pills and operation."

So, what would be the root cause?

Where was this insightful voice coming from?

She felt a strong desire to create a meaningful healing process out of this painful, potentially deathly experience but she was weak and dizzy from last night's heavy vomiting and fever. She also had been excessively drinking to ease the pain of loneliness and uncertainty for a long while now. Maybe it was the hallucination of last night's hard liquor or it was her fear of surgery that was trying to talk her out of the operation.

With this health challenge, who would know it was purpose knocking on her door?

In history, it was Viktor Frankl who first recognized that purpose is a critical component of optimal functioning, especially when challenged with the biggest adversity ever: DEATH. Viktor Frankl, a Viennese psychiatrist and a Holocaust survivor, while building a philosophy around the power of purpose and resilience, referred to Nietzsche's quote many times:

"Those who have a 'why' to live can bear almost any how." - Nietzsche

During World War II along with others, Viktor Frankl was imprisoned at concentration camps for many years. Him seeing people dying around him, including his nurse wife and his mother surviving three brutal years in various concentration camps, he always searched for a way to transform pain into purpose. At the camps, he noticed that fellow prisoners who had a sense of purpose showed greater resilience to torture and starvation. Many of the prisoners who survived the camp had someone or something to live for. Most of the prisoners who had no others, or other life outside of the camp had severe depression, boredom, and anxiety. This made him think,

"Is there a correlation between life purpose and wellness?

"How about happiness and resilience?"

"Having a purpose; can it impact health and longevity?

His real-life experiences and a system he built called "logo therapy" [26] served many. Later, he turned his life's work, his magnum opus, into a book that we all know by heart: "Man's Search for Meaning."[27]

Outcomes of his scientific observations created a quest among psychologists and medical doctors in understanding:

"What does it mean to have a purpose in life?

"How can having a sense of meaning affect our overall well-being?

"Could a meaningful life lower cholesterol levels, prevent mild dementia and even Alzheimer's?"

Quality questions through time lead us to meaningful results from dozens of surveys and analytical studies in the search for the correlation between purpose and wellness. Most world religions, spiritual paths, and many secular systems of thought have also offered guidelines for developing purpose in life. Over the past few decades, psychologists have developed many systems around

---

[26] "logotherapy" - https://www.medicalnewstoday.com/articles/320814

[27] "Man's Search for Meaning.-"https://www.oxfordscholastica.com/blog/10-psychology-books-everyone-should-read/

it, such as PIL- Purpose in Life surveys, psychological scales of well-being, and meaning in life questionnaires.

The conclusions from these tests, surveys, interviews, definitions, and meta-analyses affirm that Victor's observations around purpose and wellness were correct. There is indeed a correlation between purpose and wellness. In addition to mental, emotional, and physical health, people living with purpose were more likely to be successful than those who don't have an aim in life.

"The purpose of life is to expand our capacity to love."

Your life purpose is made up of the most important motivating goals and inspirations in your life—the reasons you get out of bed in the morning. And evolution is the process by which it is accomplished. Your purpose feeds the purpose of life and life feeds what feeds life. When you fulfill your purpose, when you become the best version of yourself; you have done your best to support evolution. The time you start living a life on purpose you are in love daily, you are grateful to all that there is, you become happy, are in peace, resilient – your nervous system gets activated in such a way that you tap more into your divine intelligence and presence.

Purpose can also direct life decisions, influence behavior, shape goals, provide direction, and generate meaning. Some people associate purpose with vocation—meaningful, satisfying work. Others find their meaning in their obligations to family or friends. Some look for meaning in spirituality or religious beliefs. Or many people may find their life's purpose clearly expressed in all of these aspects.

Past and recent research shows that people who live on purpose have these 5- five common characteristics:

1. People who live a life of purpose tend to be physically better off than those who do not. Studies done by Burton Singer and Gayle Love in 2004[28] found that highly purposeful older women had lower cholesterol and lower levels of inflammatory response than those who didn't have a purpose in life.

A study that took place in 2010 by Patricia Boyle and her colleagues at The Rush Alzheimer's Disease Center[29] found that individuals who reported higher purpose scores on cognitive tests were less likely to be diagnosed with mild cognitive impairment and even Alzheimer's. After following more than 900 elderly people at risk for dementia for seven years, they found that those with a high purpose in life were only half as likely to develop Alzheimer's than those with a lower PIL score.

Other studies as in Adam Kaplin, MD's[30] have looked at purpose in life and risk of heart attacks. Following 1500 people with cardiovascular disease for two years, researchers found that a higher baseline PIL was linked to a lower risk of a heart attack.

---

[28] Burton Singer and Gayle Love in 2004 -https://www.researchgate.net/scientific-contributions/Gayle-Dienberg-Love-39389540

[29] Patricia Boyle and her colleagues at The Rush Alzheimer's Disease Center - https://www.sciencedaily.com/releases/2012/05/120507164326.htm

[30] Adam Kaplin, MD - https://www.ncbi.nlm.nih.gov/pmc/articles/PMC4564234/

Adam who was at Yale University back then[31] focused on the interactions between mind, body and how purpose in life can directly affect health. His research reveals exciting correlations between PIL (Purpose in Life) tests and positive health outcomes. In conclusion, purpose, a sense of direction in life soothes inflammation, and lower levels of inflammatory response. Purpose protect neurons, lowers the risk of heart attacks, and lowers cholesterol levels. Purpose, a sense of direction in life reduces the risk of dementia and even Alzheimer's.

People who have a purpose in life live longer too. Dr. Dan Buettner and NIH National Institutes of Health study[32] followed people between the ages of 65 and 92 for eleven years to find a correlation between having a sense of purpose and longevity. Individuals who expressed having clear goals or a purpose lived longer and happier lives than the ones who didn't.

Later, Dr. Buettner did research with National Geographic[33] to confirm these results on longevity and purpose.

They discovered five spots in the world - Blue Zones.[34] This is where people living on purpose live an average of 90 plus years. Okinawa - Japan, Sardinia - Italy, Nicoya - Costa Rica, Ikaria - Greece, and Loma Linda - California. When they did extensive

---

[31] Dr. Adam Caplan from Yale University -
https://www.researchgate.net/publication/282038769_New_Movement_in_Neuroscie nce_A_Purpose-Driven_Life

[32] Dr. Dan Buettner and NIH National Institutes of Health -
https://www.ncbi.nlm.nih.gov/pmc/articles/PMC6125071/

[33] Dr. Buettner did research with National Geographic -
https://www.ncbi.nlm.nih.gov/pmc/articles/PMC6125071/

[34] Blue Zones - https://www.bluezones.com/about/history/

research on seven of the elderly Japanese men and women around Okinawa, they noticed that all seven had unusually high levels of DHEA in their bloodstream. DHEA[35], considered as the longevity hormone, is linked to a longer lifespan, lower cancer risk, and better memory. Interestingly, it wasn't their diet or environment that caused their bodies to make more of this miracle hormone.

What discovered was they all had an Ikigai - a reason for being, a purpose for waking up in the morning.

2. In addition to stamina and longevity, people who live lives of purpose tend to be psychologically better off than those who do not. Scientific studies find that individuals without a purpose in life are more likely to suffer from depression, boredom, loneliness, and anxiety. People who have a clear goal in life wake up happy, they are excited to live their day, have a positive outlook. They have joy no matter what, and can find humor in nearly everything. Remember that Italian movie, La vita è bella - Life is beautiful by Roberto Benigni?[36]

People living on purpose have high levels of life satisfaction. They are grateful for everything. Even in the most challenging times, they find something to be grateful for.

And studies over the past two decades, have consistently found that people who practice gratitude report fewer symptoms of illness, including depression, more optimism and happiness, stronger relationships, more generous behavior says the

---

[35] DHEA, considered as the longevity hormone, is linked to a longer lifespan, lower cancer risk, and better memory - https://professional.diabetes.org/abstract/association-dehydroepiandrosterone-insulin-sensitivity-male-adults-and-longevity-japan

[36] La vita è bella - Life is beautiful - https://www.imdb.com/title/tt0118799/

researchers at Greater Good Science Center at UC Berkeley - the epicenter for research on happiness and gratitude.[37]

3. People who have a purpose are less likely to show suicidal behavior. They are more resilient. The result of Victor Frankl's studies shows that when experiencing conflict, disaster, war, violence, or abuse, people that have a purpose in life adopt these stresses positively.[38] They tend to learn and grow from these extreme experiences. They transform pain into purpose. They have a growth mindset. A growth mindset is a belief that intelligence can be nurtured through learning and effort. Whereas, the fixed mindset believes that one's talent, intelligence, personality traits, and creativity are fixed and cannot be changed. The work of Stanford psychologist, Dr. Carol Dweck found that a growth and purpose mindset allows people to thrive during some of the most challenging times in their lives.[39]

4. People that have a clear goal in life tend to be more successful in academic and business life. Scientific studies from 2004 [40] with millennials show that having a clear purpose improves academic outcomes, persistence, and the amount of time students were willing to spend studying for tests and completing

---

[37] Greater Good Science Center at UC Berkeley-
https://greatergood.berkeley.edu/topic/purpose

[38] People who have a purpose are less likely to show suicidal behavior. They are more resilient. - https://www.ncbi.nlm.nih.gov/pmc/articles/PMC7046995/

[39] Dr. Carol Dweck found that a growth and purpose mindset allows people to thrive during some of the most challenging times in their lives - https://hbr.org/2016/01/what-having-a-growth-mindset-actually-means

[40] Scientific studies from 2004 with millennials -
https://www.researchgate.net/publication/303266473_The_millennial_generation_A_strategic_opportunity

homework. Purposeful work leads to increase in employee engagement and leads to higher scores in teamwork, grit, perseverance, passion, resilience, and self-efficiency.

5. People that have a purpose in life love to contribute, give back to their communities. They find joy in sharing their resources with their communities and the world. The more they contribute, the more meaningful experiences, coincidences, synchronicities, and joy show up in their lives. Researchers at Florida State University and Stanford found that being the giver in a relationship connected people with having a more purposeful life.[41]

We have covered a lot of scientific research on life purpose, and wellness, haven't we? Not just doctors and scientists, but also philosophers, theologians, and many ancient civilizations have asked these questions:

"Why are we here?"

"How can we have a happy, healthy, and fulfilled life?"

"What gives us a sense of meaning?"

Life's purpose has been there from the early days of human consciousness and been investigated in many different cultures. In Japanese culture, it's called "Ikigai" - the reason for being. Nicoyans long-lived residents of Costa Rica call it "Plan De Vida."

---

[41] Researchers at Florida State University and Stanford -
https://news.stanford.edu/news/2014/january/meaningful-happy-life-010114.html

Ancient Polynesians, Hawaiian, Tahitian, and Maori New Zeland cultures call it "MANA" - a supernatural life force that flows through us when we live on purpose. Interestingly, mana - meaning purpose of life, is a word rooted in ancient Greek and Hebrew, meaning "the essence of a tree – honeydew of a tree."

In Farsi, the Persian Empire used mana as a concept that brought immortality. They believed that when one or a community had strong mana, their essence would live forever. Mana was also used in Ottoman Empire, in Sufism and Kabbalah.

In the ancient books of Abrahamic religions, we can see the term Manna - bread from heaven created during the twilight of the sixth day of Creation. It is believed that people that survived the desert for 40 years without food and water; with the sunrise would be given Manna, an unseen spiritual bread. Some theologians said this ancient group of people were walking with purpose and in full faith. They had a MANA – a compelling future with a higher purpose in their life, that is why they were able to bear hunger and thirst. Nietzsche was right, "those who have a 'why' to live can bear almost any how."

By the way, do you remember the girl in the hospital with severe pain? What does she do from here? Did she get the operation and meds? Nope! She didn't know at the time but statistics from the World Health Organization showed 88% of deaths each year are due to lifestyle diseases such as obesity, diabetes, cancer, dementia, and Alzheimer's. [42] We see these

---

[42] World Health Organization showed 88% of deaths each year are due to lifestyle diseases such as obesity, diabetes, cancer, dementia, and Alzheimer's. - https://www.who.int/news-room/fact-sheets/detail/dementia

diseases when people do make bad lifestyle choices, when they're unhappy, uncertain, in fear, and pain.

"It is in your moments of decision; your destiny is shaped."

- *Tony Robbins.*

Thank God, that girl in pain made a good decision. That early morning, after signing what seemed to be 300 pages of hospital documentation, she left the hospital with the surveillance of her friends. At that moment, even though it was a risky and scary decision, she committed to self-healing through lifestyle changes. She took a leap of faith and left her job, her old life for over four months. She created a safe healing environment at her healer-nurse friend's house. After a slow-paced life, changing her lifestyle, working on her mindset, letting go of disempowering beliefs and emotions, eating healthy, studying Ayurveda, Macrobiotics, doing yoga, meditation, and spiritual practices, simply utilizing her talents on what she loves to do and her focusing on a higher purpose, she has transformed pain into purpose. Lifestyle Medicine not only saved her but also helped her to connect to her life purpose.

Extensive research over the last decades has confirmed that the vast majority of chronic symptoms can be stopped or reversed using the 4 evidence-based pillars of Lifestyle Medicine:

1. EAT WELL

• Eat mostly whole-plant-based foods

• Drink mostly water, tea, herbal teas

• Avoid risky, toxic, processed substances

2. EXERCISE MORE

• Regular fitness & strength training

• Mindful, stress-reducing exercise

3. STRESS LESS

• Let go of psychosocial stress

• Increase restorative sleep

4. LOVE MORE

• Give and receive love

• Connect with a higher purpose

• Strengthen social connections

It's no coincidence when we transform fear into love, ego into soul, let go of our selfish desires and attachments to pain and traumas of "i" instead when we focus on "we" even the word "illness" magically transforms into "wellness." At the end of the fourth month, doctors confirmed that she had no symptoms whatsoever of that bleeding cyst anymore.

That day, I learned that I was healed and that was my moment of decision; was I going to go back to my old life; bad habits, alcohol, cigarettes, working many long hours with little income in a passionless job, just surviving, or was I going to focus on my purpose - to the vision that was given to me: a happy, healthy, and fulfilled life?

Purposeful, good decisions followed, and I did choose to take the call, left the corporate world, and did set up my holistic life coaching and consulting business in Southern California. In the first year of my business, along with many other doctors in the field of Holistic Health, with Johannes R. Fisslinger too, we created 10 city festivals all around the United States called "National Yoga Month" to create awareness around yoga and health. Our vision led the US Department of Health and Wellness to officially designate September as the National Yoga Month in 2008.[43] Since then, in the States and all around the world, Yoga Month is celebrated every year in September.

That girl's courage and commitment to a purposeful path have led her to many meaningful and successful adventures all around the world. Yes, my search for meaning and purpose started in 2006 in that emergency room.

In 2010, at an event called "A Date with Destiny", it has evolved into an even higher purpose. This event is conducted by world-wide know leader, speaker, philanthropist Tony Robbins. It is a six days and six nights event where Tony assists its participants to find the answer of "What is my Life Purpose?", especially focusing on several people who were suicidal or depressed. He also provides tools to reshape our destiny and design the life of our dreams.

Date with Destiny event not only totally altered my and many others lives and it is also scientifically proven by Stanford University research doctor's[44] that through the completion of this program core rules, values, most importantly beliefs in the way that they see the world shifts and this leads them towards a happy,

---

[43] National Yoga Month - https://www.forbes.com/sites/jeannecroteau/2019/09/02/september-is-national-yoga-month--how-you-can-get-started/?sh=4b3bf3852b30

[44] Tony Robbins events - https://scienceoftonyrobbins.com/

healthy, wealthy life; lowers depression and eliminates suicidal thoughts.

Later, purpose-led me to create a system that I call "MANA Life Purpose and Wellness" which I teach at Lifestyle Prescriptions® University along with Johannes and many other trainers in the field of Lifestyle Medicine. I also had the opportunity to share this concept "MANA" on the same stage along with many world-wide known doctors, leaders, spiritual masters, scientists and many more.

So, what's the takeaway here?

I believe that purpose creates happiness and wellness. I'm a firm believer that we come to this world with our individualized purpose. We have a unique DNA of our soul. It is only when we awaken and honor this unique path that our lives flourish with true meaning.

It feels so good once we have a life purpose. Whenever we face challenges in life, we lose momentum or passion, we can go back to our purpose and all of a sudden everything soothes out and we are passionate again. When the problem, the depression, and the anxiety come in, we tend to focus on the things we cannot control. And we start to jump into the future or back into our history. All this mind chatter creates anxiety. Through realigning with our values and purpose we can tap back into wellness.

The real question is: How to find meaning through the search of it? I wish to conclude with five questions that will lead you to find your unique life purpose – your Ikigai Mana.

Answer in the wrong order and you will miss your purpose altogether. Answer in the right order and you will live with the kind of fulfillment and meaning you have been craving. Now, take a piece of paper and write down the answers to these five questions.

1. What do you love? - Write down the things that you love. What sets your heart on fire? What's most important for you?
2. What are your talents? - Write down your talents. What are you good at? What do people come to you for? Do a personal SWOT analysis.[45]
3. What does the world need? - How would you like to help a world problem? Look at the people around you and the world. What can you do to help? Is it hunger, poverty, education problems, climate change, peace, good health, and wellbeing?
4. What can you get paid or rewarded for? – How would you like to do to earn or be rewarded to support your desired lifestyle?
5. And as the fifth element add MANA to the equation: Design a life on purpose aligned with your values, create daily, monthly, yearly rituals that fulfills your soul. Obtain a sustainable living doing what you love while utilizing your talents to help and contribute to something bigger than you. That is your unique life purpose.

Rest is taking action with SMART (Specific, Measurable, Action-oriented, Realistic, Timed) goals towards that compelling

---

[45] SWOT analysis - https://www.investopedia.com/terms/s/swot.asp

future. Maybe even add an – ER (Evaluated, Reviewed) at the end of it for smarter goals for a healthy, wealthy, fulfilled life.

As Nelson Mandela wisely said,

"Action without vision is only passing time. Vision without action is daydreaming. But vision with action can change the world."

And so can your purpose! So, start with your why. Search it, find it and start living it!

Chapter Twenty-One

Dr. M.I. Yamani - #1 Medical Error: Failure To Diagnose and Value-Based-Care.

Mohammad Ilyas Yamani, MD, MMM is a Board Certified, Internal Medicine Physician, CEO, a value-based primary care provider, specializing in lifestyle medicine. Ilyas still sees patients daily and manages three offices, acting as CEO and Medical Director of All Care Medical. ↗ allcare4u.com

I'm in primary care but we call it value based care. Like in any other industry now in the United States of America, the businesses are going towards value creation. And in our case, we want to create value for patients.

Although this is so obvious, it is strange in the medical industry that we are here to create value for patients.

Traditionally so far, unfortunately, medicine revolves around providers such as hospitals, doctors, their schedule, their timing, are they covered, everything is around those institutions.

Finally, the pendulum is shifting towards value creation for the patient, which is, in short, number one, to improve patient outcome results and number two, lower the cost.

As you know, cost is a major issue for healthcare in the United States, compared to any other country per patient per year, the cost of care is two to three times more than any other. France is number two, which is almost $5000 to $6000 a year per patient lower than the US. The cost is an issue and I happen to be on the management side, on the process improvement side, on the clinical operations side.

I own my own businesses also, but I own what we call a management service organization. We manage financial risk on people's lives. Our goal is to figure out how to really improve the outcome and this search introduced me to mitigate risk through a lifestyle modification, almost 13 years ago.

That's how I found Doctor Dean Ornish, and since then I've been his student and follow his recommendations. My Centre in Florida is one of the two centers of Doctor Dean Ornish and we practice lifestyle modification.

What I have done is I have merged regular primary care and lifestyle modification in one place which is only possible because my contractual agreement based on value-based care.

Therefore, we get paid if the patient's outcome is better, and we don't get paid if the outcome is no different or worse.

So basically, I have burned my bridges. Fortunately, we have done wonderfully both financially as well as the patient's outcome.

For today's topic, I wanted to discuss the one fundamental issue in having an improved outcome and unfortunately, the industry generally does not pay attention to that. Generally speaking, in the industry, when we talk about medical errors, we talk about what happened in the hospitals; how many infections in the hospital, how many patients fell down, how many get pneumonia and they try to go after those kinds of sentinel events.

Sentinel events are described after the fact that the patient is already in the hospital or after the fact that the patient is already on medications. In short, we are looking for errors in the treatment. But after today's topic, if you don't get anything from it, but if you just take home this one point, that more than failure of treatment, the error in overall medical care is the failure to diagnose.

There is no solid definition of what medical error is or how you would define that. I found a wonderful definition is the use of the wrong plan to reach an aim in medical care and it starts from the moment a patient comes into the office and we start talking to the patient. That's where we kind of get to know patients and diagnose them for the first time. For those of us listening here, they do their regular medical care, those people who are the listeners, those who are practicing Lifestyle Medicine in any shape or form for them, whatever I'm going to say today they're going to say 'of course we know that's the issue'.

But for those who are on the fence or those like me, who are mainly mainstream medical doctors or providers and they are on the fence and they are not sure how to incorporate Lifestyle Medicine and Root-Cause Analysis, which is what we are trying to educate patients about, at Lifestyle Prescriptions® University[46]. They will see the point I'm trying to make.

What happens is in a regular medical practice, primary care is the key. That's where it all starts. So, we have a huge responsibility because once you put a diagnosis in the chart of the patient that becomes the genetic code of that patient. The patient carries that record forever. It's part of their permanent record. It's like a physician is biased by looking at the past medical history. If somebody has made the diagnosis of congestive heart failure, the

---

[46] Lifestyle Prescriptions® University www.lifestyleprescriptions.tv

next physician who's seeing the patient is not going to question that.

Most likely, we just take it okay, this is CHF. Let's design the treatment accordingly. So, making the first diagnosis is the utmost important because the whole system decides how we assign funding to patient care based on diagnosis.

A lot of people think making a diagnosis is a medical art. No, it is not.

It is a socio-economic definition; it is a construct that we have given to society. It is not really about health; it is about the socio-economic division of the whole thing. So, once the diagnosis is made, now the whole socio-economic system will revolve around it.

Understand that your first diagnosis that you make is going to drive the outcome and the cost.

I have given a lot of examples and the research that has been done so far. Instead, one of the famous reports from the IOM, in 1998, is called, "To Err is Human." A lot of references are there and historically, even though it was in 1998, it is still very relevant. If you are in medical management, and if you are on the financial side of things, this is one of the Holy Grails. This is one of the fundamental research projects that we refer to.

In that report, it was said 98,000 deaths in the United States every year were attributed to medical error. There is another, a John Hopkins study was done in 2016. And it was published in the British Medical Journal, they said no, it is 251,000 deaths every year.

251,000 deaths every year because of medical error. That makes it the third leading cause of death after cancer and after heart disease.

I just want you to see that this is the outcome, and the cost, those kinds of events are not even registered.

I'll give you a little example; if the patient comes in with abdominal pain, and the funny statistic says that a primary care physician gets seven minutes to diagnose a case - seven minutes in the first visit.

An average primary care physician interrupts patients in the first six seconds, as soon as the patient starts opening their mouth they are interrupted. It's an average number, a national number but imagine by doing that, we just slap a medication in place.

For example, a very famous, very common medication that we prescribe is called proton pump inhibitors, PPI, like Omeprazole, Pantoprazole. Anybody who just said, 'oh, I'm having indigestion or abdominal discomfort,' that's it, you're going to get PPI.

The side effects of PPI, cause impairment of the acid production and the whole physiology of the gut changes.

Now this patient can go with nausea, vomiting, or may end up in the emergency room. At the emergency room they are going to do CT scans, do a whole battery of tests, sometimes endoscopy and everything. So, imagine the costs if we would have taken better history through the method that we learn here at Lifestyle Prescriptions® University.

278

We would know that there are a lot of other things going on with this patient and a PPI was not needed. So, you put a stop to at least $15,000 costs by just listening to that patient for a little longer.

I know Johannes, how you go back and forth to educate us to take the history of the patient and it doesn't take a long time. It's not like you have to sit down in a therapy session for hours and hours to get to know the patient.

When we evaluate our patients with Root-Cause Analysis based on Organ-Mind-Brain Anatomy™, and know where the root causes it's amazing how quickly we can help.

Basically, diagnosis is the foundation and something on which all healthcare services and treatments rest. Another report back in 2005 from the same Institute of Medicine, which shows how to improve diagnosis identified that failure to diagnose is the most underestimated cause of medical error.

We talk about treatment options, we talk about other things, but we have not emphasized that it is underestimated how we don't emphasize on the wrong diagnosis. Incorrect diagnosis, some statistics; in inpatients, 5% of patients suffer from diagnostic error, outpatients it is 17%, I'm sure these percentages are in fact worse, there is a lot of misdiagnoses going on there in medical care.

So, what happens when something wrong happens, a sentinel event happens; somebody dies or somebody has complications which are very severe, what happens? Those events are reportable. Institutions, offices and doctors have to report that as an adverse event. Those events also get reported to a data bank, and it's called National Practitioner Data Bank, and future licensing is attached to that data bank, this is a very solid structure, physicians are very aware of it.

We know that we don't want our name or any adverse case attached to you going into the data bank. I just took some reports from that data bank; 28% of all reported cases are related to misdiagnosis, not making correct the diagnosis. 28%!

That comes down to almost $39 billion of cost.

I am sure that these reports are being reported to them. There are a lot of sentinel events happening which are not being reported. So, this number is maybe a minute fraction, but I just wanted to make it tangible. So, I wanted us to know that not only is that bad for patient care, but it is costly for the society, for any society to survive like that.

There was another report from Project HOPE where they talked about individual physician decision making. What happens is that if you're a medical student, you're going to be taught about how to decide, protocols are there and how the system is designed to make the diagnosis. Nobody emphasizes taking the information from patients or understanding how to do the patient's history and physical.

Basically, in a physical, we should ask the patient, how is your day? This is like knowing your patient and it is fundamental to our way of prescribing care in Lifestyle Medicine.

The patient-physician interaction as in the report that Project HOPE compiled, they found that patient-physician interaction emerged as a major contributor to the diagnosis failure, no surprise for us, but these are all reported things.

So why are professionals and the people who are running the show, not in the national news? It is one of the big things. The reason is because nobody wants to open that can of worms, because they don't know how to close it. It is not because the data is not there. The data is there. It is very strong data, but it has not been talked about because it is very hard to really tackle that issue right now.

It is unprofessional clinical behavior to admission behavior or ignoring the patient's knowledge or what kind of factors indicate an issue and it will become clear if we're going to talk to the patient the way we learn here at LPU. The harm is obvious and the explanations, the thing is, at the Lifestyle Prescription University, fundamentally you're learning that root cause analysis is important. We talk about; stress management, emotional awareness, knowing the belief system, knowing what they're doing on a daily basis and how much they know about the organs, mind and body. As a healer, a provider, you have that knowledge and you're sitting in front of a patient, it's very hard to miss the diagnosis.

There are two things about the whole industry. One is how you are managing the whole system, which is called delivery of care.

For example, we have decided that this is medical care, but how are you going to provide or deliver that care to the patient, to the population - it's called a delivery system. The second is how you interact as the provider when the patient is in the room, what kind of method are you using to interact with the patient?

Our delivery system is also referred to as, 'fee for service'. This means if I'm going to see the patient, I'm going to get paid.

If I'm going to do the procedure, I'm going to get paid. If I'm going to prescribe the pill, I'm going to get paid. It is called interaction-based care like event-based care. When we bill Medicare for all this coding system, that coding system depicts that an encounter happened. So as a physician, if I'm a businessman, which I am, but I'm going to make money only when there is an interaction, when there is a face-to-face thing.

In terms of incentive, it is easy to understand that I make more money if I do more procedures.

Whereas, value-based care, now the government and Medicare is saying please improve the outcome. Ensure patients are happy; patients are healthy, that they are not asking us what to do to get there.

However, we, the practitioners - myself, working alongside Harvard Medical doctors - have collectively devised a definition. So instead of calling a disease like diabetes or chronic renal failure, we call it a medical condition, like if somebody had a stroke that patient will fall more, that patient will be incontinent, and that patient will have other issues. We therefore conglomerate that medical condition as one. We then collect the data on those patients because the data is an important factor and we make those patients a part of a community and we assign team members.

This allows us to 'go upstream' and try to prevent any issues 'upstream'. The physician is only one team member in that, you have a social worker, the social worker will go home, find out what's going on with the patient. Then a nurse practitioner will evaluate, home visits are included and office visits are available should the patient need it. Instead of calling a treatment we call it intervention. It doesn't mean a pill. It doesn't mean a procedure.

It also means a Lifestyle Medicine Health Coach, that's part of it. The whole team, until that patient - God forbid - needs to go to the hospital. We have the whole team to work with the patient as if the patient is in the hospital, we're not leaving them alone.

42% of patients in hospitals are lonely and if there's no pill to act on your body when you're lonely. I mean, it's kind of a simple thing we understand here in this forum, you take care of those patients until - God forbid - palliative care or nursing home or hospice. That's called value. We get paid by keeping those patients happy and healthy and out of critical illnesses. That's value-based care in a nutshell.

We need to provide; we need to create those providers who are into value-based care and institutions like Harvard at their gain. One funny thing about these leaders, I talked to them and they all know it, they know in their deep hearts and soul, that that's where the problem is.

It's just the system is an 800-pound gorilla, it's hard to move it. But we need to push them a bit more, we need more people to participate and we can pull it through in our lifetimes.

Chapter Twenty-Two

Dr. Kevin Chan - Secrets to successful Lifestyle Medicine Practice

Kevin Chan DO, MS, MMM, PCEO, FASA, FAIHM, FAAMFM is a board-certified lipidologist, owner of Pineapple Health in Phoenix providing expert care for over 20 years. Dr. Chan is an integrative-holistic physician who focuses on total health and especially heart attack and stroke Prevention ↗ pineapplehealth.org

When I first became a doctor a long time ago, I thought being a doctor was more like making people happy. But as I practice more and more over the next 20 years, I come to realize that more and more physicians, many of them are becoming more frustrated.

And why is that? I wondered.

It can be said that it is because of the system. The culture of the medical institution is not conducive to a good patient or compassionate patient care. We could always blame the forever-profit-driven nature of Big Pharma and insurance companies as well as the forever-power-seeking nature of the government. But the reality is many patients are not happy with what they're getting.

And more than 50% of physicians have reported burnouts.

What shall we do then? Well, you might say perhaps I should start my practice. If I do my own business, maybe I can download a few forms on the internet, or maybe I can subscribe to a few services, have my practice and stay independent, an autonomist.

Then maybe I can stay away from the handcuffs and the bureaucracy of healthcare panelists and I'll become less burnout.

But we quickly find out that by having our own business, it's going to be as difficult, as challenging, as frustrating as anything else, because running the business for ourselves has its challenges and obstacles.

Focusing on integrative Lifestyle Medicine, of course, functional holistic, that's only half of the equation. The other half is, how to implement them.

I offer Lifestyle Medicine and knowing that for the past 20 years, I have come to realize that there is a set of core principles that I can use in my journeys through my trials and errors. I came to realize that many of these principles, possibly thousands of years old, apply to the success of our own business. Many of which are quite applicable to life coaching or even, of course, lifestyle and health coaching. Hence, three key areas have been identified to be so fundamental,

Strategic principle number one is exploration and exploitation. Please note, it's not stated as exploration "versus" exploitation. Studies show that maybe no more than 2% of the world's companies are doing well - both exploitation and exploration.

Many experts believe that the reason why most practices and companies fail is that they're either doing too much of one or the other, too much exploration, or too much exploitation. For example, imagine you have a gold mine.

What you do naturally is to protect the gold mine, treat it like a fortress, defend it, exploit it, and try to extract as much value as possible and get the most out of it. This continues until a point of diminishing returns is reached when there is less and less gold to be extracted and more and more people coming in, trying to get a piece of the action. And then you realized that the pie was getting smaller and smaller and smaller until you had to say to yourself, you know what? It's time to explore like a ship going out on a journey, to find out where the next gold mine is.

In general, exploitation usually focuses more on immediate or near-future needs, focuses more on linear thinking, focuses on process improvement, quality control, etc. Typical strategies include locking up the resources, captivating customers or patients, and taking advantage of the economy of scale. If in your business you ask the question, how am I going to offer as many services as I can to as many patients as possible in my practice?

That's exploitation. On the other hand, exploration is more focused on future needs. It uses a different way of thinking, more adaptive, more learning, more experimenting, and more innovation. The strategies would be like, I want to go to the next market earlier. How about creating a whole new category through blue ocean strategies? But the big mission that is going to change the whole world soon is called the MTP - Massive Transformative Purposes.

You might also ask, how am I going to bring in new patients and what type of new service line should I start? Once again, a successful company, that lasts a long time can do both - exploitation and exploration.

In general, they spend 70% of their resources on exploitation, on growing their core business. While spending 30% of their resources on exploring, on emerging, and on new markets. But that's one more thing to consider – timing.

The timing here means when should something be done? In general, when we start a new business venture, of course, we're going to focus more on exploring until the business becomes more mature then, of course, we can start to exploit more.

But what else? Depending on how stable and how dynamic the landscape is. If the landscape or the environment of the marketplace is more volatile, uncertain, complex, and ambiguous, then know that we are much more likely to have to fall back on exploration earlier. So in summary, a successful company does both in a balanced way of exploring and exploiting pretty much in a loop that goes on over and over again, and that exactly leads to the second principle which is to improve our position over time, slowly, through unity and focus.

Most people would love to have overnight success without realizing that most overnight successes are preceded by many smaller steps over time. Those smaller steps usually can stem on an average of over 10 years. These small steps represent the reiteration of the loop of exploitation, exploration. Over time, that allows you to quickly experiment and find out what you have done right and what you can improve on to get your BHAG - Big, Hairy, Audacious Goal.

The problem though with a BHAG sometimes is that's, it's great and can give you a general direction of where you want to be, but BHAG could be far, distant, and challenging. In time, you may lose focus, motivation, not inspired anymore, and may even lose direction. So it's important to come back and focus on these smaller steps to get to the BHAG in a more timely fashion.

Knowing that the path is rarely going to be straight or linear. It is almost always going to be convoluted, torturous, or even a zigzag pattern.

Studies show that for those fast-growing hi-tech companies, they found that the average age of the founder is 45 years old. Those who are in their fifties have twice the success as those founders who are in their thirties. So 'yay', remember success comes later in life, be patient, even though you are trying to get to your BHAG sooner. And once again, what are the benefits of a smaller step experimentation model?

- Number one, it uses fewer resources, it saves costs, and therefore it has lesser risk even your mistakes.
- Number two, because a smaller step, a smaller scale, is very similar to the SMART goal that we use for our Lifestyle Medicine coaching patients, these small steps generally have a shorter cycle time.

A shorter cycle time allows you to access your outcomes sooner and so that you can study your KPI faster. KPI stands for Key Performance Indicator, and also allows you to be rewarded sooner. The sooner you can be rewarded, the better you can stay focused, motivated, and inspired to continue the journey to your BHAG.

However, the most important reason for having this smaller step experimentation approach is to allow you to identify a niche or depending on where you come from, a niche segment. But why is that important? Isn't it true that one can just hang shingle somewhere, and start seeing everyone who walks through the door? Isn't it true that the best way to grow this practice is to see everyone? That may be true decades ago, but today, when the barriers to entry have been lowered, when we serve and we're trying to serve everyone, that way, we are not serving everyone well. We are now competing with everyone on every front. When competing in every front then we are defending everywhere. To defend everywhere would mean using up our limited resources everywhere, and by that, we become weak everywhere. In essence, we end up spreading ourselves too thin. So the purpose of having a niche segment allows you to dominate a smaller market space and "allows" (that's the keyword) you to scale and also to achieve what we call 'Top of Mind' mentality. You want your patient to remember what you're good at.

Once again, the benefit of doing the smaller step model is to allow us to go to our BHAG in a timelier manner. And the purpose of doing the niche segment is to allow us to scale and also achieve top of mind. But to do that, we need two more factors: unity and focus. What does that mean? Unity is a group of people having a shared mission at a given moment in time. Focus is defined as the same group of people doing a task at a given point in space. So unity and focus is essentially a time-space alignment, which allows you to generate power. For example, imagine you want to launch a rocket and of course, you want the rocket to go up. Well, how are you going to position the thrusters? Are they all going to be in different directions? No, you want all the thrusters in alignment, in one direction in a given moment of space and time, so that the rocket can launch up, not going just everywhere. Therefore remember, unity and focus give you power, which leads to the third strategic principle, which is strength and weakness.

What exactly is strength? Strength is a form of excellence. But remember, when you are excellent in something, it is also deviance from the norm. Every time you deviate from the norm, you are subject to external pressure to make you conform back to the norm, which makes you weak. True strength is a strategic process, product or service fit for the critical desire of your clients, customers, or patients in such a way that your strength becomes so effective that can make your weaknesses irrelevant. In other words, you can be so good at what you do that allows you to suck in other areas. You've got to be good at your core competence. And by the way, if your bathroom is clogged, please fix it, even though you may be one of the top practitioners in your field.

Now, it might be argued, isn't it true that you always improve your weakness? Well, other than your core competence, other areas, when you're trying to improve everything, everything becomes more average. And you're just becoming your competition, not differentiated from your competition. So remember that trying to improve our weaknesses is diluting our strength.

Another example is having been an osteopathic physician for over 20 years. Back then, I was worried that there was some stigma attached to being an osteopathic doctor. But I positioned myself specifically to those patients who are interested in integrative, holistic, functional, and Lifestyle Medicine. Now, 20 years later, my practice is exclusive. Many come to me because they do not like the mediocre doctoring experience that they get from conventional allopathic physicians. Another example is if you are a member of the IFM, they use a slogan that "we change the way we do medicine and the medicine that we do." I use that phrase to constantly remind my patients that as an osteopathic physician, I am always here to do health.

Remember, what makes you different, makes you wonderful and what makes you weak, makes you strong. So, turn your weakness into strength.

Following the three principles could make a very big difference. Not just for you but the patient because, when a patient comes, you are not just interested in fixing the symptoms, you want to go after the cause. And one of the common things in conventional medicine is that we simply focus on the outcome of, let's say, aging, which is a generation. But with lifestyle medicine, we're not just focusing on the outcome; we are focusing on the process. If we can focus on the process of aging, for example, we can tremendously affect the outcome and that's exactly what we do in Lifestyle Medicine. Not just focusing on the outcome, but focusing on the process. When we spend time looking at the root cause, we can completely change the course of patient health. That's a huge difference.

Again, using the three principles can serve as a foundation for making several changes in medicine overall.

For example, using the first model. You need to protect your core, then slowly. 70% of what you should be doing is to protect your core business. That could be insurance or that could be conventional medicine. And then slowly, use 30% of your resources to start to explore what you should do in your lifestyle. Looking at the second principle, we don't ever say to our colleagues, "Let's drop everything and start tomorrow!" Some can afford to do that but most don't. We may all have different experiences but we don't want to risk our livelihood or walk up to our family and say we will quit our job and then suddenly do it the next day. So, you get to abandon your existing position slowly, but move to the new position quickly.

So once again, exploit continuously 70% and explore 30% over time. And of course, this is not to say you want to achieve success overnight. It takes time to slowly build up your position over time. This is an incremental change. The advice is, leave your current position slowly and start something new early, and quickly. Then explore what is right for you and continuing with that is being able to identify a niche, because if you try to do everything, then you're going to have to use up so many resources, and then you're going to feel it is all too overwhelming and you can't do it. That's why, when you explore, explore what you are good at and focus on that niche. Not only does it take fewer resources, but you can also become an expert.

You could do this and be able to have what is called a top-of-mind mentality, followed by looking at what your weakness is.

Oftentimes, what you think is your weakness can be turned into your strength.

Finally, this has been a summary of the three key areas or principles which are considered to be most fundamental, at least, to be successful in lifestyle medicine.

- Number one, exploitation and exploration.
- Number two, focusing on smaller steps that allow you to get to your BHAG and don't forget, unity and focus.
- Number three, turn your weakness into strength.

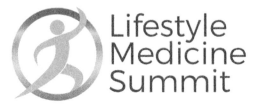

Register for our upcoming global
Lifestyle Medicine Summit at
www.lifestylemedicine.io

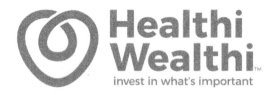

Shouldn't you get "PAID" living healthier, happier, longer, and richer?

Get your Personal 24/7 Health Coach
or build your Health Coaching practice.

Join our Global Movement,
redeem your RXHEAL reward tokens,
and read the book "HealthiWealthi™".

www.healthiwealthi.io.

Printed in Great Britain
by Amazon